Psychiatric Services for Addicted Patients

A Task Force Report of the
American Psychiatric Association

The American Psychiatric Association Task Force on Psychiatric Services for Addicted Patients

Sheila B. Blume, M.D. (Chairperson)
Myron Belfer, M.D.
Donald J. Gill, M.D.
Walter Ling, M.D.
Peggy S. Stephens, M.D.

Psychiatric Services for Addicted Patients

A Task Force Report of the American Psychiatric Association

Published by the American Psychiatric Association
Washington, DC

Note. The authors have worked to ensure that all information in this book concerning drug dosages, schedules, and routes of administration is accurate as of the time of publication and consistent with standards set by the U. S. Food and Drug Administration and the general medical community. As medical research and practice advance, however, therapeutic standards may change. For this reason and because human and mechanical errors sometimes occur, we recommend that readers follow the advice of a physician who is directly involved in their care or the care of a member of their family.

The findings, opinions, and conclusions of this report do not necessarily represent the views of the officers, trustees, all members of the task force, or all members of the American Psychiatric Association. The views expressed are those of the authors of the individual chapters. Task force reports are considered a substantive contribution of the ongoing analysis and evaluation of problems, programs, issues, and practices in a given area of concern.

American Psychiatric Association
1400 K Street, N.W., Washington, DC   20005

Library of Congress Cataloging-in-Publication Data
American Psychiatric Association
    Psychiatric services for addicted patients : task force report of
the American Psychiatric Association. — 1st ed.
        p.   cm. — (Task force report)
    Includes bibliographical references and index.
    ISBN 0-89042-276-1
        1. Substance abuse—Treatment—United States.   2. Substance abuse—
Treatment—United States—Finance.   3. Substance abuse—Economic
aspects—United States.   I. Title.   II. Series: Task force report
(American Psychiatric Association)
    DNLM: 1. Substance Dependence—therapy.   2. Substance Dependence—
psychology.   3. Mental Health Services—United States.
4. Financing, Government—United States.   W1 TA82 1995 / WM 270
A51065p 1995]
RC564.65.A46   1995
362.29′18′0973—dc20
DNLM/DLC
for Library of Congress   95-3162
                                                                                      CIP

British Library Cataloguing in Publication Data
A CIP record is available from the British Library.

Contents

Contributors

Myron Belfer, M.D.
Professor of Psychiatry, Department of Social Medicine, Harvard Medical School, Boston, Massachusetts

Sheila B. Blume, M.D.
Medical Director, Alcoholism, Chemical Dependency, and Compulsive Gambling Programs, and Director, The South Oaks Institute of Alcoholism and Addictive Behavior Studies, South Oaks Hospital, Amityville; and Clinical Professor of Psychiatry, State University of New York at Stony Brook, Stony Brook, New York

Donald J. Gill, M.D.
Director, Substance Abuse Programs, Pennsylvania Hospital/Institute of Penn Hospital; and Clinical Associate in Psychiatry, University of Pennsylvania Medical School, Philadelphia, Pennsylvania

Walter Ling, M.D.
Professor of Psychiatry and Chief of Substance Abuse Treatment Programs, University of California, Los Angeles; Director, Los Angeles Addiction Treatment Research Center; and Medical Director, Matric Center, Los Angeles, California

Peggy S. Stephens, M.D.
Clinical Director of Adult, Dual Diagnosis, and Adolescent Acute Programs and Outpatient Services, Charter of Jefferson Hospital, Jeffersonville, Indiana; and Instructor, University of Louisville, Department of Psychiatry and Behavioral Sciences, Louisville, Kentucky

Summary

Addiction has been of great interest to American medicine and psychiatry since the time of Benjamin Rush. However, both medical and social (including criminal justice) conceptualizations of addictive disorders and their treatment have changed markedly during the 19th and 20th centuries. Perhaps in the treatment of no other group of disorders has there been such a tension between medical and criminal justice approaches.

During the past several decades, the federal government has assumed a leadership role in supporting research into the treatment of addictive disorders and the development of treatment services. This was largely accomplished through the development of the National Institute on Alcohol Abuse and Alcoholism (NIAAA), the National Institute on Drug Abuse (NIDA), and the Substance Abuse and Mental Health Services Administration (SAMHSA).

Organized psychiatry has also been active in advocating for improvement in research and treatment for addictive disorders. This task force report is one product of psychiatry's increased attention to these problems.

In 1990, the American Psychiatric Association (APA), acknowledging the major role of addiction treatment within psychiatry, established the Council on Addiction Psychiatry. Then, in March 1991, the Task Force on Psychiatric Services for Addicted Patients was appointed with the charge of producing a monograph that would accomplish the following:

1. Define psychiatrists' current roles and practices in the treatment of substance-dependent patients in relationship to that of other practitioners, with particular attention to issues such as dual diagnosis, methadone treatment, and detoxification

2. Develop suggestions for appropriate funding mechanisms for the payment of addicted patients' treatment in the context of managed care and indemnity benefit programs
3. Examine issues related to the funding of public sector programs, including funding of Department of Veterans Affairs programs, block grant funding of state and city programs, as well as funding of voluntary treatment programs within and outside the criminal justice system

The original task force report, completed in the summer of 1994, reflected the current state of addiction treatment and provided recommendations for improving these services in the future. That monograph is reproduced in this book.

This book is organized into four sections. In Chapter 1, "Introduction," the history of American psychiatry's interest in disorders of addiction and the development of the current network of addiction treatment services are reviewed. For the last half century, official position statements of the American Medical Association and other medical organizations have encouraged humane treatment for patients with addictions, as well as research, training, and insurance coverage for addiction treatment. Addictive disorders are characterized as complex biopsychosocial entities, closely related to many physical diseases (e.g., acquired immunodeficiency syndrome [AIDS]) and medical complications (e.g., cirrhosis of the liver); they are further characterized by high mortality rates. Also in Chapter 1, data from the Epidemiologic Catchment Area Study (Regier et al. 1990) are briefly reviewed, documenting the common occurrence of addictive disorders, their onset in adolescence or early adulthood, and their comorbidity with other psychiatric disorders. Finally, the role of the psychiatrist in addiction treatment is summarized, with a discussion of its similarities to the patient care role assumed by the federally designated primary care specialists.

In Chapter 2, "Services for Addicted Patients," a snapshot of the current addiction treatment system is provided, with a description of the services provided in general medical settings, psychiatric hospitals, freestanding residential facilities, and private practice and other outpatient settings. The goals of treatment, types of therapies employed, and role of the psychiatrist are discussed for each setting. The chapter ends with a look at the size, scope, and other characteristics (e.g., ownership, occupancy rates) of the current treatment system, based on the latest available SAMHSA data.

In Chapter 3, "Support for Addiction Treatment," the economics of the treatment system are explored: the costs of addictive diseases to American society and the costs and sources of support for their treatment. Although estimates of societal cost vary with the methodology used, in the United States, the total cost related to addictive disorders is well over $100 billion dollars annually. The total amount spent on treatment is also difficult to estimate because of the multiple sources of financing involved, but adds up to several billion dollars. In Chapter 3, current information on cost-benefit ratios, cost-effectiveness of treatment, and cost offsets associated with addiction treatment are also reviewed, with the conclusion that investment in treatment makes good economic sense. Other issues addressed include insurance for addiction treatment (including benefit utilization), cost-containment measures, and the role of private and public insurance systems (e.g., Medicare, Medicaid, Civilian Health and Medical Program of the Uniformed Services). Direct public support for treatment is discussed, including that provided through federal block grant programs, the Department of Veterans Affairs, the U. S. military, and the Indian Health Service. Finally, other sources of support, such as charitable contributions, asset seizures, and dedicated taxes, are summarized.

In Chapter 4, "Needs of the Addiction Treatment System," the range of system modifications and resource allocations needed to bring high quality, cost-effective treatment to addicted patients and their families is considered. These needs range from improving data collection and treatment research to increasing community involvement and the application of current research findings. The roles of health care reform and the direct and indirect public support of treatment in the future are discussed, with recommendations for including the treatment of addiction in any system of health care reform on a basis equal to that provided for other diseases.

Reference

Regier D, Farmer ME, Rae DS, et al: Comorbidity of mental disorders with alcohol and other drug abuses. JAMA 264:2511–2518, 1990

Chapter 1

Introduction

Historical Overview

Although alcohol and other drug dependencies have been recognized as important medical problems throughout the nation's history, the development of adequate systems for preventing and treating these diseases has proved a daunting task. The modern disease concept of addictive disorders owes much to the work of Benjamin Rush, the father of American psychiatry (Rush 1785/1943). In his 1785 treatise on "An Inquiry Into the Effects of Ardent Spirits Upon the Human Body and Mind," Rush described inebriety as a disease and outlined principles for its treatment. In addition, Rush was the first to articulate the idea of addiction to a drug, characterizing inebriety as an addiction to "spirituous liquors" (Levine 1978). He also made the first epidemiological estimate of the extent of alcohol dependence (4,000 deaths per year in a population of less than 6 million) and compared the disease with slow suicide (Rush 1976).

During the 19th century, physicians routinely treated alcoholism and other addictions. A medically directed State Inebriate Asylum was established in Binghamton, New York in 1864. The Association for the Study of Inebriety, an organization of physicians interested in alcoholism, was founded in 1870. The organization's journal, the *Quarterly Journal of Inebriety,* was published for 37 years (1876–1913). Opiate dependence was increasingly recognized during the latter half of the 19th century, especially after the invention of the hypodermic needle in 1843 permitted more concentrated administration of opiates (Lewis and Zinberg 1964). Heroin was introduced in 1898 and was used in the treatment of alcohol dependence, as was cocaine.

Interest in treating addictive disorders waned as first the temperance movement promoting prohibition (Lender and Martin 1982) and then the criminal justice approach to the control of other drug problems (Gerstein and Harwood 1990) competed with medical approaches. By the post-prohibition era, there was little interest in addiction treatment. Many hospitals had policies against admitting alcoholic patients to their wards. Physicians routinely treated the physical and mental complications of addictive disorders, such as trauma, hepatic cirrhosis, delirium tremens, and Wernicke-Korsakoff's syndrome, but few took an interest in treating the underlying addiction. Treatment of these complications was well known to generate frustration among health professionals who watched their patients leave the hospital improved, only to return in a worse condition after resuming their substance use. It was this observation by Dr. Norman Joliffe at Bellevue Hospital in New York in 1935 that formed one of the roots of the modern "alcoholism movement" (Keller and Doria 1991). His frustration in treating the gastrointestinal manifestations of alcoholism led to curiosity about the underlying alcohol addiction, which in turn led to the formation of a committee to review the literature and encourage research into the causes and treatment of alcoholism. This activity stimulated the organization of the Yale Center of Alcohol Studies in the late 1930s (Lender and Martin 1982). At almost the same time, the Public Health Service opened its narcotic treatment hospitals in Lexington, Kentucky (1935) and Fort Worth, Texas (1938). These facilities became the first centers for the systematic study and treatment of opiate dependence (Pickens and Fletcher 1991).

A third important influence on the development of renewed interest in addiction treatment was the birth of Alcoholics Anonymous (AA) in 1935. By adopting a disease concept into its philosophy and by demonstrating that large numbers of men and women formerly considered hopeless alcoholics could recover, AA focused both lay and professional attention on the problem of alcoholism.

Psychiatrists have been interested in addictions since Rush's time. A number of conceptual approaches have been proposed, generally in the context of underlying psychopathology and understanding alcoholism or other drug addiction as a symptom of some other disorder. For example, in 1937, an expert in the field of alcoholism wrote, "Alcohol addiction is a symptom rather than a disease. . . . There is always an underlying personality disorder evidenced by obvious maladjustment, neurotic character traits, emotional immaturity, or infantilism" (Knight 1937). Psychiatrists often attempted to treat addiction by searching out underlying psychic conflicts or uncovering early traumata. The American Psychiatric Association's (APA's) first *Diagnostic and Statistical Manual of Mental Disorders* (DSM-I), published in 1952, did not permit an independent diagnosis of alcohol addiction if an underlying disorder was present.

As the interest in addictions once again grew within both general medicine and psychiatry, the concept of addictive disorders as primary diseases requiring specific treatment grew as well. Later editions of the APA's *Diagnostic and Statistical Manual* provided independent diagnostic categories for addictive disorders, at the same time that they recognized the frequency of the comorbidity of these diseases with other psychiatric disorders.

Position of Organized Medicine

It is of interest that various medical organizations have seen fit to develop policy statements on addiction treatment. In 1956, the American Medical Association (AMA) published a position paper urging physicians and hospitals to admit and treat alcoholic patients, applying the term *illness* to alcoholism. In 1966, the AMA reaffirmed this position and included in its policy statement a reference to the disease concept of alcoholism. This position was again reaffirmed in 1988 (American Medical Association 1992). In a 1987 policy declaration, the AMA stated that both alcohol dependence and other drug dependencies were diseases that constituted a legitimate part of medical practice (American Medical Association 1992).

In 1965, the APA published a position statement entitled "Concerning Responsibility of Psychiatrists and Other Physicians for Alcohol Problems." This thoughtful statement urged psychiatrists and other physicians to obtain appropriate education and take an active role in managing alcohol problems. It decried discrimination against alcoholic patients by both general and psychiatric hospitals, and encouraged the inclusion of alcoholism treatment in health insurance plans. The APA established a separate Council on Addiction Psychiatry in 1990, recognizing the increasing importance of addiction treatment in psychiatric practice.

The American Hospital Association also adopted a strong position in 1957, encouraging general hospitals not to discriminate against alcoholic patients and to develop alcoholism services (American Hospital Association 1957).

In 1954, the American Society of Addiction Medicine was founded (then named the New York Medical Society on Alcoholism). This organization of 3,100 physicians attained a seat in the AMA House of Delegates in 1988. In 1982, about one-third of the society's members were psychiatrists (Galanter et al. 1982); as of 1994, 37.6% were psychiatrists (J. F. Callahan, Executive Vice-President ASAM, personal communication, 1994). The American Academy of Psychiatrists in Alcoholism and Addictions was founded in 1985 and as of 1994 had over 1,000 members. Both organizations have been advocates for the establishment of high-quality, accessible addiction treatment.

In 1991, the Group for the Advancement of Psychiatry, through its Committee on Alcoholism and the Addictions, published a position paper in which it was stated that all psychiatrists "should possess expertise in the recognition, assessment and treatment of substance use disorders" (p. 1292).

The number and exhortative nature of these medical policy statements reflect the social stigma attached to alcoholic patients and individuals addicted to other substances in 20th century American society. Both the lay public and the general medical profession have tended to look on the substance-addicted patient's woes as self-inflicted and therefore as less worthy of attention and sympathy than the illnesses of others. Both organized medicine and lay interest groups have been working actively to reverse these negative attitudes for the past 50 years.

Features of Addictive Disorders

The substance-related disorders, as described in DSM-IV (American Psychiatric Association 1994), include abuse and dependence on specific substances along with a diagnostic category for polysubstance dependence (dependence on more than one substance if there is no clear-cut predominant drug). These diagnostic entities represent separate disorders that may coexist with a variety of other psychiatric disorders, including personality disorders.

The addictive disorders themselves are complex because they are influenced by genetic, familial, psychological, and sociocultural factors. Intervention measures often involve not only the substance-dependent patient, but family members of several generations and other members of the patient's extended social network. Employee-assistance–based intervention techniques may include supervisors, friends, and co-workers. Court-based intervention may involve judges, probation or parole officers, and others. School-based intervention may include parents, teachers, and school counselors. Prevention measures include policies related to the manufacturing, distribution, and prescription of psychoactive drugs; the production and marketing of alcoholic beverages and tobacco products; and the interdiction of the illegal drug trade, in addition to the more traditional educational, refusal technique, and self-esteem building approaches.

More often than is the case with other psychiatric disorders, substance use disorders are associated with physiological changes and medical complications. Drug overdoses and withdrawal states may represent medical emergencies. Sequelae of long-term, heavy drinking (e.g., pancreatitis, cirrhosis, infections, peripheral neuritis, various cancers) complicate alcohol dependence treatment. Endocarditis and other forms of sepsis complicate the course of intravenous drug dependence, as does the spread of the infectious agents responsible for acquired immunodeficiency syndrome (AIDS) and hepatitis B and C. Drug-addicted individuals, especially those infected with the human immunodeficiency virus (HIV), have also shown a recent increase in active pulmonary tuberculosis, including infection with bacterial strains resistant to antituberculous therapeutic drugs. Tobacco use, usually accompanied by nicotine dependence, is associated with a wide variety of cardiovascular and pulmonary disorders and malignancies and was implicated in approximately 419,000 deaths in 1990 ("Cigarette Smoking" 1993).

Individuals with addictive disorders have high rates of mortality from several causes. In addition to accidental overdose, trauma, and the physical complications mentioned above, suicide is often related to alcohol and other drug abuse-dependence. For example, in their 2- to 20-year follow-up study of nearly 4,000 male and 1,000 female adult patients who had been hospitalized for alcoholism in Stockholm, Sweden, Lindberg and Agren (1988) found that mortality risk was elevated by a factor of 3 for the men and by a factor of 5.2 for the women. Significant excess mortality was found for hepatic cirrhosis, pancreatitis, tuberculosis, pneumonia, ischemic heart disease, suicide, violent death, and digestive system, and hepatic, lung, and breast cancers. The substance use disorders are also a factor in adolescent mortality, particularly in relationship to accidents and homicides. Likewise, both alcohol and other drug use disorders have been found common among adolescents who commit suicide, especially males (D. Shaffer, M. Gould, P. Fisher, et al.: "Psychiatric Diagnosis in Child and Adolescent Suicide," submitted for publication, 1994).

In addition to the direct physical damage to the user, psychoactive substances may also act as teratogens when consumed during pregnancy. Birth defects—including those resulting from fetal alcohol syndrome and other fetal alcohol effects; nicotine-, opiate-, cocaine-, or cannabis-related growth retardation; and a variety of other structural and behavioral abnormalities—have been associated with prenatal substance use (Hoegerman et al. 1990).

Epidemiology of Addictive Disorders

Substance use disorders are common in the general public and likely to be associated with other psychiatric disorders. In the Epidemiologic Catchment Area (ECA) Study, involving more than 20,000 adults in the general public (including those in institutions), Regier et al. (1990) found a lifetime prevalence for alcohol abuse-dependence of 13.5% (making it the most common of all diagnoses) and a lifetime prevalence of other drug abuse-dependence of 6.1%. The median age at onset for alcohol abuse-dependence was 21 years and, for other drug abuse-dependence, 19 years (Christie et al. 1988). However, late-onset cases, particularly of alcohol dependence and prescription drug dependence, are not unusual.

The authors of the ECA Study also found that 45% of those with alcohol abuse-dependence and 72% of those with other drug abuse-dependence had an additional alcohol- or drug-related or psychiatric disorder. For those with an alcohol- or drug-related disorder, the odds of having a comorbid disorder of another substance-related category were increased by a factor of 7. A lifetime diagnosis of alcohol abuse-dependence increased the chances of having a non–substance-related mental disorder by a factor of 2.3. For those with other drug abuse-dependence, the odds ratio for having a non–substance-related mental disorder was 4.5 compared with that of adults in the general population with no substance use disorder (Regier et al. 1990).

As expected, prevalence rates for addictive disorders among the 1.3% of the total population found to be residing in institutional settings were found to be higher than those for the population at large. Among psychiatric hospital patients, 39.6% had a lifetime prevalence of psychoactive substance abuse-dependence (34.1% with alcohol abuse-dependence and 16.1% with other drug abuse-dependence). Among prison populations, 72% had a lifetime prevalence of an addictive disorder, with alcohol abuse-dependence in 56.2% and other drug abuse-dependence in 53.7%. In nursing home populations, 14.3% had a lifetime prevalence of alcohol or other drug use disorders (Regier et al. 1990).

The 1-year prevalence for any substance use disorder in the general population was found to be 9.5%, with 7.4% meeting criteria for alcohol abuse-dependence and 3.1% other drug abuse-dependence. About 1% had both and 3.3% of the adult population (about a third of those with addictive disorders) met diagnostic criteria for both substance abuse-dependence and a non–substance-related psychiatric disorder during the year (Regier et al. 1993).

All of the above epidemiological data exclude the diagnosis of nicotine dependence, a major addictive disorder affecting millions of Americans that is especially prevalent among those with other substance abuse-dependence. Various studies of clinical populations in treatment for psychoactive substance dependence have found that about 80% of such subjects are also regular heavy users of tobacco, and presumably dependent. As of 1991, approximately 27% of American adults in the general population reported themselves as current cigarette smokers (Department of Health and Human Services 1991). The majority are presumably physically dependent on nicotine (Jarvik and Schneider 1992).

One of the most serious deficiencies in psychiatry's knowledge of epidemiology is the lack of data regarding substance use disorders in child and adolescent populations. A "youth ECA" study is sorely needed.

Development of the Service Network in the United States

Developments in the 1960s and 1970s

The current network of specialty treatment services for addicted patients developed at varying rates and in different ways in different parts of the country, leading to a markedly uneven distribution of facilities and treatment capacity (Institute of Medicine 1990).

Several treatment approaches to the substance-dependent population developed in parallel during the 1960s and 1970s. One was the residential therapeutic community model, staffed mostly by nonprofessional, recovering substance-addicted individuals and pioneered by Synanon in 1958 (Pickens et al. 1991). Synanon was based in part on the philosophy of AA and in part on the model of the psychiatric therapeutic community (Gerstein and Harwood 1990). The therapeutic community model was subsequently implemented and developed in both freestanding facilities and prisons. A second advance was the introduction of methadone maintenance treatment for opiate-addicted individuals (Dole and Nyswander 1965). During the late 1960s and 1970s, outpatient methadone maintenance clinics were established around the country, guided and controlled by detailed government regulation.

These program models grew side-by-side with inpatient drug detoxification and outpatient nonmethadone treatment programs (e.g., drug-free programs). In addition, Narcotics Anonymous (NA), a self-help fellowship adapted from the 12-step method of AA, was founded in 1953 and spread rapidly (Narcotics Anonymous 1982). This fellowship is widely recommended as an adjunct to treatment, along with the companion fellowship for friends and family members, Nar-Anon.

Although these treatment programs for drug-addicted (most often heroin-addicted) patients were being established, a parallel and sometimes intersecting alcoholism treatment system was also being developed. Early outpatient programs were based on a clinic model, developed at the Yale Center of Alcohol Studies in the 1940s and 1950s, that combined medical care, counseling, referral to AA, and, at times, disulfiram (Antabuse) treatment (Lender and Martin 1982). Inpatient medical detoxification units were also established to treat serious alcohol withdrawal. Later on, as many states adopted legislation to decriminalize public intoxication during the 1970s, "social setting detoxes" or "sobering-up stations" were developed to replace jail-based "drunk tanks," (Institute of Medicine 1990; Lender and Martin 1982).

During the 1950s to 1970s, residential alcoholism treatment units were being established that combined services by professional medical and mental health personnel, alcoholism counseling (often provided by specially trained recovering alcoholics or family members of alcoholics), and AA meetings (Institute of Medicine 1990). The residential alcoholism facilities stressed family involvement, where possible, and a continuum of care. These units, often referred to as *Minnesota Model programs* because their roots were traced to three Minnesota programs that began in the 1950s (Willmar State Hospital, the Hazelden Foundation, and the Johnson Institute [Institute of Medicine 1990]), were established in freestanding facilities as well as in public and private hospitals. Although some of the programs varied from the original plan, they all retained its major elements. In addition, a number of longer term community residences, called *quarterway houses, halfway houses,* or *recovery homes,* grew to accommodate those alcoholic patients who lacked families or social supports during early recovery.

The development of the alcoholism and other drug addiction treatment systems was greatly enhanced following the passage of several federal measures that facilitated funding for addiction treatment. The Narcotic Addiction Rehabilitation Act of 1966 authorized community-based treatment for substance-addicted individuals released from incarceration. A 1968 amendment to the Community Mental Health Centers Act supported alcoholism and other drug treatment within community mental health centers (Institute of Medicine 1990).

A major step in federal efforts to fight substance addiction occurred in 1970 with the passage of the Comprehensive Alcohol Abuse and Alcoholism Prevention Treatment and Rehabilitation Act, which established the National Institute on Alcohol Abuse and Alcoholism (NIAAA) (Lender and Martin 1982). This was followed by the establishment of the National Institute on Drug Abuse (NIDA), which, with NIAAA and the National Institute of Mental Health (NIMH), came under the auspices of the Alcohol, Drug Abuse and Mental Health Administration (ADAMHA). These institutes helped develop and implement new program models (e.g., em-

ployee assistance programs), provided funding for demonstration programs of new treatments, funded and conducted treatment-relevant research, and provided funding to the states in the form of *formula grants*
(later reorganized as *block grants*) to aid in the establishment of alcohol
and drug treatment networks (Gerstein and Harwood 1990; Institute of
Medicine 1990). The organization of this federal system was changed in
1992, with NIMH, NIDA, and NIAAA moving to the National Institutes of
Health, and the Substance Abuse and Mental Health Services Administration (SAMHSA) replacing ADAMHA and assuming administrative responsibility for the block grants and direct program funding. SAMHSA
incorporates the Center for Substance Abuse Prevention (formerly Office
of Substance Abuse Prevention), the Center for Substance Abuse Treatment (formerly Office of Treatment Improvement), and the new Center for
Mental Health Services.

Contemporary Developments

Although federal funds were appropriated separately to support alcoholism
and other drug programs, and although much of the development of these
programs was accomplished in separate facilities, in the late 1970s and
1980s a movement began to combine alcoholism and other addiction
treatment. This trend had its roots in inpatient alcoholism units as patients
with multiple addictions began to be the rule rather than the exception.
Nicotine dependence had always been a major accompaniment of alcoholism. However, sedative-, marijuana-, stimulant-, and, to some extent, opi-
ate-dependence diagnoses became more and more frequent. The
alcoholism treatment model became extended to a chemical dependency
model, with the 12-step approach of AA and NA being applied to all of the
substance use disorders. This was particularly true in the private, for-profit
sector that expanded rapidly during the 1980s, paid for by improved health
insurance coverage of alcohol- and drug-use disorders for employed individuals and their families.

These developments led to what the Institute of Medicine Committee
for the Substance Abuse Coverage Study (Gerstein and Harwood 1990)
called *the two-tiered structure* of the treatment system—that is, a division
between public, drug-focused programs and private, chemical dependency–focused programs. For example, in 1987, the public tier, serving

mostly indigent patients, provided 636,000 drug dependence (i.e., non-alcohol dependence) treatment episodes, whereas the private sector, mainly through chemical dependency programs, provided 212,000 drug dependence treatment episodes to working class and middle- and upper-class cocaine- and marijuana-dependent patients (Gerstein and Harwood 1990). This public-private division of services is also evident in alcoholism treatment, with certain facilities (e.g., social setting detoxes) serving indigent populations and others treating only those with insurance coverage.

In addition to the two-tier nature of contemporary addiction treatment, the present network of services is characterized by a marked unevenness in distribution. Many regions of the country entirely lack sufficient services. In others, inpatient programs may be available but community residential programs, halfway houses, and partial hospital services may be lacking, leading to an overreliance on inpatient care. In rural areas, outpatient and family services may be geographically inaccessible, whereas in population centers access may be limited by overcrowding and waiting lists. For example, whereas in 1987 the national average treatment capacity for inpatient-residential alcoholism rehabilitation services was 0.21 per thousand individuals, the capacity in various states and territories varied from 0.49 in the District of Columbia, 0.48 in Alaska, and 0.43 in Minnesota to 0.09 in West Virginia, 0.10 in South Carolina, and 0.11 in Georgia, Illinois, and Indiana. Likewise, the outpatient alcoholism treatment capacity varied from 0.2 treatment "slots" per thousand in Alabama to 3.34 per thousand in Colorado (Institute of Medicine 1990).

The above data are derived from federal studies of treatment in specialty addiction treatment units as identified by the responsible state agencies. However, data from the ECA Study (Regier et al. 1990) collected between 1980 and 1985 indicated that many substance-addicted individuals received their care outside of the specialty mental health-addictive disorders system (Regier et al. 1990). During a 1-year period, 23.6% of adults with a diagnosable addictive disorder (22% of all adults with alcohol abuse-dependence, 30% of all adults with drug abuse-dependence) received some help during that year. Only 11.2% received help in the specialty mental health-addictive disorders sector, whereas 9.9% were treated in the general medical sector and 4.4% in the voluntary sector (e.g., self-help, family, friends). Less than half of those who received help in the voluntary sector (2% of those with addictive disorders) attended self-help sessions during the year. Not surprisingly, those with comorbid mental and addictive disorders had greater treatment rates (37.4% received services, with 20.6% receiving care in the specialty mental health-addictive disorders sector, 16.3% in the general medical sector, and 11.4% in the voluntary sector). Most of the treatment for these dual-diagnosis cases was given in mental health rather than addiction-specific facilities (Regier et al. 1990).

Unfortunately, comparable treatment utilization data are not available for children and adolescents. Also of interest would be utilization data for gay and lesbian populations, as some studies have indicated that these individuals show a high rate of addictive disorders (Cabaj 1992). In addition, there appear to be gender-related differences in where patients receive their treatment. For example, results from a recent study of a Northern California county (Weisner and Schmidt 1992) indicated that female problem drinkers were more likely than males to obtain care in health care settings that were not alcohol specific and to delay treatment until problems were more severe. Women with alcoholic problems in particular were likely to be treated in mental health settings.

The tendency for addicted patients to seek help in general medical and mental health settings should be kept in mind in reviewing the material about specialty addiction treatment in Chapter 2 (in which the components, magnitude, and characteristics of the current addiction treatment system are addressed) and Chapter 3. To some degree, the use of treatment services other than addiction-specific treatment programs may be a function of maldistribution, lack of addiction treatment insurance coverage, long waiting lists at public programs, and other barriers to treatment; however, the reasons for usage patterns among various groups await study.

Role of the Psychiatrist in Addiction Treatment

Because of its unusual developmental history, the present addiction treatment network is notable for the multidisciplinary nature of its treatment approaches, in which medical-surgical and psychiatric evaluation are combined with treatment through psychoeducation, counseling by credentialed addiction counselors (many of whom are in recovery from their own addictive disorders), and self-help through lay fellowships. The medical leadership of these programs has also been multidisciplinary, with the role of medical director in organized addiction programs assumed by a psychiatrist, an internist, a family physician, or a pediatrician trained and skilled in addiction medicine. Depending on the nature of the program and the training and background of the medical director, other medical specialists fulfill varying full-time, part-time, or consulting roles in the treatment process.

Despite these variances, the psychiatrist plays a critical role in the care of addicted patients (American Psychiatric Association 1965; Group for the Advancement of Psychiatry 1991). For many addictive disorder patients treated in the mental health system and in private psychiatric practice, the psychiatrist is routinely assigned primary medical responsibility, with a role similar to that of a federally designated primary care specialist (Khantzian 1988). As such, the psychiatrist coordinates all aspects of clinical care, acts as a "gatekeeper" for referral to other services, interacts with the patient's family, and provides ongoing monitoring of the patient's overall condition. The psychiatrist can also evaluate and respond to problems experienced by these patients with regulation of affect, self-esteem, interpersonal relationships, and various aspects of behavior during a long-term therapeutic relationship (Khantzian 1988).

A 1988–1989 APA survey (Dorwart et al. 1992) of over 19,000 practicing psychiatrists indicated that psychoactive substance abusing or dependent patients made up slightly more than 10% of those psychiatrists' average caseload (defined as all patients seen at least once in the past month). When asked to indicate their areas of special interest in psychiatry, 34% of respondents mentioned alcohol abuse and 33.4% mentioned drug abuse among their designated areas of concern (American Psychiatric Association, Office of Survey Designs and Analysis, personal communication, December 1992).

A 1991 nationwide survey of drug and alcoholism treatment units (Department of Health and Human Services 1992a) identified 4,654 psychiatrists employed full- and part-time in the 9,057 treatment units surveyed. In a 1991 report to Congress (Department of Health and Human Services 1992b), the Bureau of Health Professions of the Health Resources and Services Administration estimated that about 5,400 psychiatrists provided services (2,900 as directly employees and 2,500 on a contractual basis) to patients in alcohol and other drug treatment services, based on data from the Drug Services Research Survey.

The many roles of psychiatrists in the care of addicted patients in the various types and settings of treatment are discussed in Chapter 2, along with a general description of the organization, goals, and operation of these treatment services.

References

American Hospital Association: Policy on Alcoholism. Hospitals 31:106, 1957

American Medical Association: Recommendations for the admission of alcoholics to general hospitals. JAMA 162:750, 1956

American Medical Association: Proceedings of the House of Delegates, 20th clinical convention, Las Vegas, NE, November 1966, pp 184–189

American Medical Association: Policy 95.983—Drug Dependencies as Diseases: Policy Compendium. American Medical Association, Chicago, IL, 1992

American Psychiatric Association: Diagnostic and Statistical Manual of Mental Disorders, 1st Edition. Washington, DC, American Psychiatric Association, 1952

American Psychiatric Association: Position statement: concerning responsibility of psychiatrists and other physicians for alcohol problems. Am J Psychiatry 122:454–456, 1965

American Psychiatric Association: Diagnostic and Statistical Manual of Mental Disorders, 4th Edition. Washington, DC, American Psychiatric Association, 1994

Cabaj RP: Substance abuse in the gay and lesbian community, in Substance Abuse: A Comprehensive Textbook. Edited by Lowinson JH, Ruiz P, Millman R. Baltimore, MD, Williams & Wilkins, 1992, pp 852–860

Christie KA, Burke JD, Regier DA, et al: Epidemiologic evidence for early onset of mental disorders and higher risk of drug abuse in young adults. Am J Psychiatry 145:971–975 1988

Cigarette smoking–attributable mortality and years of potential life lost—United States, 1990. JAMA 270:1408–1413, 1993

Department of Health and Human Services: National Household Survey on Drug Abuse: Population Estimates 1991 (DHHS Publ No ADM-92-1887). Washington, DC, US Government Printing Office, 1991

Department of Health and Human Services: Highlights From the 1991 National Drug and Alcoholism Treatment Unit Survey (NDATUS). Washington, DC, Department of Health and Human Services, 1992a

Department of Health and Human Services: Health Personnel in The United States: Eighth Report to Congress 1991. (DHHS Publ No HRS-P-OD-92-1). Washington, DC, US Government Printing Office, 1992b

Dole VP, Nyswander MA: Medical treatment for diacetylmorphine (heroin) addiction. JAMA 193:646–650, 1965

Dorwart RA, Chartock LR, Dial T, et al: A national study of psychiatrists' professional activities. Am J Psychiatry 149:1499–1505, 1992

Galanter M, Blume SB, Bissell L: Physicians in alcoholism: a study of current status and future needs. Alcohol Clin Exp Res 7:389–392, 1982

Gerstein DR, Harwood HJ (eds): Treating Drug Problems, Vol 1. Washington, DC, National Academy Press, 1990

Group for the Advancement of Psychiatry: Substance abuse disorders: a psychiatric priority. Am J Psychiatry 148:1291–1300, 1991

Hoegerman G, Wilson C, Thurmond E, et al: Drug-exposed neonates. West J Med (special issue) 152:559–564, 1990

Institute of Medicine: Broadening the Base of Treatment for Alcohol Problems. Washington, DC, American Psychiatric Press, 1990

Jarvik ME, Schneider NG: Nicotine, in Substance Abuse: A Comprehensive Textbook. Edited by Lowinson JH, Ruiz P, Millman R. Baltimore, MD, Williams & Wilkins, 1992, pp 334–356

Keller M, Doria J: On defining alcoholism. Alcohol Health Res World 15:253–259, 1991

Khantzian EJ: The primary care therapist and patient needs in substance abuse treatment. Am J Drug Alcohol Abuse 14:159–167, 1988

Knight RP: The dynamics and treatment of alcohol addiction. Bull Menninger Clin 1:233–250, 1937

Lender ME, Martin JK (eds): Drinking in America: A History. New York, Free Press, 1982

Levine HG: The discovery of addiction. J Stud Alcohol 39:143–174, 1978

Lewis DC, Zinberg NE: Narcotic usage: a historical perspective on a difficult medical problem. N Engl J Med 270:1045–1052, 1964

Lindberg S, Agren G: Mortality among male and female hospitalized alcoholics in Stockholm 1962–1983. Br J Addict 83:1193–1200, 1988

Narcotics Anonymous. Van Nuys, CA, World Service Office, 1982

Pickens RW, Fletcher BW: Overview of treatment issues, in Improving Drug Abuse Treatment. Edited by Pickens RW, Leukefield CG, Schuster CR. National Institute of Drug Abuse Research Monograph 106 (DHHS Publ No ADM-91-1754). Washington, DC, US Government Printing Office, 1991, pp 1–19

Pickens RW, Leukefield CG, Schuster CR (eds): Improving Drug Abuse Treatment. National Institute of Drug Abuse Research Monograph 106 (DHHS Publ No ADM-91-1754). Washington, DC, US Government Printing Office, 1991

Regier DA, Farmer ME, Rae DS: Comorbidity of mental disorders with alcohol and other drug abuse. JAMA 264:2511–2518, 1990

Regier DA, Narrow WE, Rae DS: The de facto U. S. mental and addictive disorders service system: epidemiologic catchment area prospective 1-year prevalence rates of disorders and services. Arch Gen Psychiatry 50:85–94, 1993

Rush B: An inquiry into the effects of ardent spirits upon the human body and mind, with an account of the means of preventing and of the remedies for curing them (1785). Reprinted in Keller M: Classics of the alcohol literature. Q J Studies Alcohol 4:321–341, 1943

Rush B: An alcoholism classic: an inquiry into the effects of ardent spirits on the human body and mind. Alcohol Health and Research World, Summer 1976, pp 7–9

Weisner C, Schmidt L: Gender disparities in treatment for alcohol problems. JAMA 268:1872–1876, 1992

Chapter 2

Services for Addicted Patients

Specialized treatment of substance use disorders takes place in a variety of settings. There are two general goals of addiction treatment: to eliminate the abuse of substances and to promote the patient's physical, psychological, and social well-being. The clinician's initial task is to conduct a comprehensive diagnostic assessment to discern the necessary level of care and then engage the patient and family in making a commitment to the recommended treatment plan. Recognition of several potentially confounding factors (e.g., denial, organicity, dishonesty, enabling behaviors, stigma, hopelessness, transference and countertransference issues) will assist in accomplishing this critical initial task (Frances and Miller 1991; Gallant 1987). Pharmacological treatments are specific to the drug of abuse and immediate problem (e.g., overdose, withdrawal). Psychosocial modalities, including individual, group, and family therapies, are adapted to addiction treatment (e.g., Blume 1984; Zimberg et al. 1985). Successful treatment fosters hope, psychological change, and emotional maturation, which, in turn, consolidate recovery, decrease the risk of relapse, and possibly promote emotional growth beyond the individual's level of premorbid functioning (Group for the Advancement of Psychiatry 1991).

Programs in General Medical Settings

There have been numerous studies of the prevalence of substance use disorders in patients admitted to general hospitals. Prevalence rates for alcohol abuse-dependence vary from about 15% to 50% from private to public institutions (Beresford et al. 1984). In their 1989 study, Moore et al.

found that 25% or more of general hospital medical-surgical and psychiatric inpatients who were formally screened for alcoholism using the Michigan Alcohol Screening Test (Selzer 1971) or CAGE test (Ewing 1984) were found to be alcoholic. Screening of patients in general hospital outpatient clinics for alcohol abuse-dependence have yielded rates of 5%–36% (Buchsbaum et al. 1991; Cleary et al. 1988). In addition, significant rates of alcohol abuse-dependence are regularly encountered in emergency rooms, trauma centers, and general medical clinics.

Other substance use disorders are also found within the boundaries of the general hospital. Emergency rooms and obstetric-gynecology services have been impacted by the wave of cocaine use in the 1980s. Opiate dependence can be discovered in patients presenting to emergency rooms, trauma centers, and particularly pain clinics. Benzodiazepine dependence can be found in patients presenting to general medical clinics and nursing homes or intermediate care facilities.

Despite the well-documented prevalence of these disorders, researchers have found that clinical personnel are not likely to diagnose or treat addictive disorders directly. Detection rates vary among different general hospital services. Moore et al.'s (1989) comparison of these services indicated that it was in psychiatry services that patients' alcoholism was most likely to be discovered, through the use of formal screening instruments. Although medical and neurology staff detected alcoholism in more than one-quarter of their alcoholic patients, diagnostic rates were lower on surgical or obstetric-gynecology services. The proficiency of psychiatrists in making the diagnosis of alcoholism would be beneficial if extended to other clinical services within the general hospital.

This is not to say that physicians do not have a sense of the prevalence of substance use disorders. When, in one survey (Orleans et al. 1985), primary care physicians were asked to report the common problems seen in their practice, about two-thirds of them named alcohol abuse-dependence as one of them. Yet this general perception does not seem to translate into specific behaviors in actual practice. For example, in one general medical clinic, there was no mention of alcoholism in the medical records of about half of the patients who screened positive for alcoholism in a research study (Buchsbaum et al. 1991). In another family practice center studied, less than 10% of patients with histories of alcoholism were so charted (Leckman et al. 1984).

Where physicians do intervene with alcoholic patients identified as such on clinical services, such interventions have proven effective in reducing posthospital alcohol abuse (Moore et al. 1989). This is true in emergency rooms as well as inpatient services (Gentilello 1989).

Some services have become attuned to the value of screening and early diagnosis and intervention. In a 1987 study of trauma centers (where about half of the patients seen had abused alcohol), Persson and Magnusson reported that about half of the centers indicated they did screen for alcohol abuse-dependence, although less than one-third had personnel with specific training in alcoholism.

More typically, medical-surgical service staff do not pursue screening or intervention. When a somatic disease is likely to have been caused by alcohol, alcohol abuse-dependence may be diagnosed. However, even when this diagnosis is recorded, at times no attempt to refer the patient to alcoholism treatment is made. Other alcoholic patients are neither diagnosed as being alcoholic nor referred for intervention. In their study of automobile accident patients treated in an emergency room, Chang and Astrachan (1988) showed that not a single patient was referred for alcohol abuse-dependence treatment.

A similar pattern is found regarding individuals with other substance use disorders. Individuals who use intravenous drugs present to surgical services with cellulitis, open wounds, and fractures, and to medical services with infection or delirium. Yet, discharge diagnoses grossly underrepresent the prevalence of substance use disorders and do not reflect adequate intervention.

Screening Programs

Although there is a striking prevalence of substance use disorders in medical settings, detection rates continue to be unimpressive. Intervention methods are promising, but are unlikely to occur if the diagnosis is missed. Furthermore, the responses of psychiatrists have differed from one facility to another.

Some psychiatry departments have helped in the detection process by making available, encouraging implementation of, or directly implementing screening tests or structured interviews. These detection efforts have seldom been hospitalwide but instead have focused on services that treat patients with anticipated high prevalence rates of addiction, such as emergency rooms or gastroenterology services. When detection efforts are hospitalwide, they may include providing patients with written statements of hospital policies toward alcohol-drug issues or descriptions of available services. Closed-circuit television channels for patients can provide similar information to patients at their bedside, using films that address detection, clinical services, or available social supports. Administration of hospitalwide laboratory screening tests, either direct chemical tests of urine or indirect screening tests (e.g., serum gamma glutamyl transferase, blood chemistry profiles), are useful but more likely to encounter resistance.

When testing is more focused, certain services may screen for specific substances. The gastroenterology service is an area where a higher yield might be expected for alcohol-related problems. Direct laboratory tests for alcohol abuse are likely to be helpful only shortly after admission, whereas questionnaire screening (e.g., the Michigan Alcohol Screening Test [Selzer 1971], the CAGE test [Ewing 1984]) can be instituted at any time. The recent high incidence of cocaine effects in newborns has prompted obstetric departments to consider urine screening in perinatal clinics. This has opened the door for psychiatric liaison in the development of educational programs for staff and patients as well as on-the-spot consultation services. Emergency services require broader screenings and more rapid consultation.

Consultation and Liaison

Consultation or liaison services may be provided by a solo psychiatrist in a small hospital, although multidisciplinary teams are more customary in large teaching hospitals. Relationships with the departments receiving liaison services are usually organized by discipline or by function. In services organized by discipline, physicians communicate with physicians, nurses with nurses, and so on. In this model, the psychiatrist performs the clinical examination, communicates the findings to the appropriate physician, and develops clinical policies with department heads. Social workers may communicate with a patient's family and other agencies, nurses may educate patients about the effects of substance use on the diseased organ or fetus, and addiction counselors may develop referral relationships with Alcoholics Anonymous (AA), Narcotics Anonymous (NA), or other similar self-support groups. In services organized by function, specific team members may be assigned to provide clinical evaluation, education, counseling, or referrals based on their training, skills, and experience rather than on their formal degree. Beyond providing clinical supervision, the degree of a psychiatrist's involvement in this model depends on his or her personal investment and experience.

The direct, clinical, consultation service provided to a patient by a psychiatrist-consultant is usually reimbursable and so puts little demand on hospital or department budgets. In contrast, liaison services are provided to a unit, department, or clinical program rather than to an individual patient. Liaison services are therefore much more difficult to fund but appear to have better results than pure consultation models. Their value lies in providing an ongoing relationship in education, improving case finding, and promoting bedside counseling.

The previously described gap between physicians' relatively high awareness of addictive disorders as major problems and the low rates of actual detection or intervention provided to individual patients is also seen among psychiatric consultants. Burton et al. (1991) documented that a psychiatrist-consultant is likely to spend less time initially with a patient presenting with a substance use disorder than one presenting with another psychiatric diagnosis. In addition, follow-up visits by the psychiatrist-consultant are likely to be fewer in number. Only slightly over half of the patients in Burton et al.'s study actually received referrals for aftercare. These findings further substantiate the need for additional education and training. The development of the field of addiction psychiatry should increase the profession's proficiency in these matters.

Services in Psychiatric Hospitals

The need to provide addiction services for psychiatric patients becomes apparent when the frequency of substance use disorders is studied in psychiatric populations. Lifetime prevalence rates of substance use disorders are consistently higher in psychiatric populations than in the general population (Regier et al. 1990; Scheier and Siris 1987). At the time of admission to a psychiatric inpatient service, the rates of these disorders seems to be about 20% and can be much higher (Bunt et al. 1990; Mezzich et al. 1989; Whitemarsh et al. 1986).

With rates as high as 20% or more, evaluations of substance use should be a regular part of any psychiatric admission procedure. In addition to history taking, clinical interview, and physical examination, a number of screening instruments can be used to detect substance use: pen and paper screening tests, detection of addictive substances in body fluids, or indirect laboratory measures (e.g., the liver profile).

Early detection has many advantages to the functioning of a psychiatric hospital. Substance use disorders can contribute to the evolution of certain symptom presentations (Pulver et al. 1989). For example, the impulsiveness, secrecy, minimizing, denial, lack of self-care, and perceptual distortions that are common in patients with substance use disorders can increase the rate of development of these phenomena in connection with other psychiatric disorders, thereby increasing both management problems and the patient's risk for hospitalization. The presentation of these symptoms on admission can also skew the initial diagnostic impression. In addition, the risk of suicide is higher when substance abuse–dependence is present (Winokur and Black 1987).

The presence of a substance use disorder increases the difficulties psychiatric patients commonly have in developing a therapeutic relationship (Galanter et al. 1988). Noncompliance with treatment plans is also a common consequence. Morbidity rates and treatment outcomes are adversely affected. Thus, when the hospital has not focused on addictive disorder evaluation from the outset, the costs can be high.

After the evaluation stage, there are several issues to be weighed. The first is the risk of withdrawal from the substance and the management of any withdrawal symptoms. Mortality risks are paramount in withdrawal from alcohol or sedative dependence; in both cases, an adequate sedative replacement is necessary. This may require creative management of other coexisting psychiatric disorders. Pharmacotherapy considerations are complicated by both the substances abused and the combinations of psychiatric diagnoses.

Psychosocial interventions that are aimed at addictive disorders can enhance the smooth functioning of a psychiatric unit. Creating an atmosphere of openness in the discussion of substance use can be helpful. Although their feelings of shame can block patients from volunteering a history of addiction, staff attitudes can foster (or, on the other hand, further impede) openness on these issues. Covert substance use by patients can confound the staff's understanding of current treatment unit events. Discussion of substance use and abuse in psychoeducational presentations, community meetings, or small groups can improve the overall well-being of the unit.

When substance abuse-dependence is clearly a part of the clinical problem, the introduction of traditional treatments for substance use disorders is indicated. These can be delivered in general psychiatric settings or in a unit or section where patients with similar diagnoses are grouped (Crumley 1990; also, see section on specialized inpatient programs, below).

AA and other 12-step groups are valuable services to have available for all patients in a psychiatric hospital. Patients with severe psychopathology (e.g., some schizophrenic patients) do not integrate well into typical AA meetings (Galanter et al. 1988). There are meetings specifically designed for these patients (e.g., "double trouble," Mentally Ill Substance Abuser groups). The process of these meetings tends to be more directive, the content is more concrete, and the value of psychotropic drugs (as distinct from the addicting drugs) is accepted.

Specialized Inpatient Programs

The most intensive level of care—inpatient treatment—can be provided in a specialized unit of a general or psychiatric hospital or in a freestanding facility. Such units may specialize in the care of adolescents or adults. Generally accepted indications for inpatient care include the presence of suicide risk factors, especially recent losses, feelings of hopelessness, and lack of self-preservation efforts; medical complications; actual or anticipated severe withdrawal; comorbid psychiatric illness; chronicity of addiction, particularly if multiple substances are involved; failed outpatient treatment; and lack of social support (Alterman et al. 1991; American Society of Addiction Medicine 1991; Frances and Franklin 1989; Gallant 1987; Group for the Advancement of Psychiatry 1991; Weiss and Stephens 1992).

The major goals of the first few days of treatment are medical and psychiatric evaluation, stabilization, and detoxification to prevent severe medical sequelae. As the patient is stabilized, he or she is gradually engaged in the treatment process with the specific goals of

✦ Eliminating the patient's substance abuse
✦ Enhancing the patient's knowledge of addiction
✦ Developing the patient's understanding and recognition of the progression and consequences of his or her disorder
✦ Improving the patient's self-esteem and coping skills
✦ Developing the patient's awareness about and management strategies for addressing factors that can trigger major relapses
✦ Introducing the patient to the 12-step recovery philosophy and integrating him or her into the recovery community
✦ Developing a continuing care plan for the patient

Treatment modalities may include

✦ Individual psychotherapy to understand and focus on those issues that will enhance psychological function
✦ Addiction counseling to address the patient's needs to establish a strong recovery plan
✦ Group psychotherapies to provide group support and feedback
✦ Psychoeducation to teach about addiction as a disease, the biopsychosocial consequences and medical complications of addiction, the 12-step philosophy, nutrition, the potential for infection with the human immunodeficiency virus (HIV), and other aspects of physical and mental health
✦ Attendance at either AA or NA meetings or both to gain recovery skills and support from the recovery community
✦ Behavioral therapies
✦ Pastoral counseling to address spiritual needs
✦ Art or expressive therapy to provide alternative modes of expression
✦ Educational services for adolescents and adults
✦ Vocational rehabilitation counseling to improve job performance
✦ Occupational or recreational therapy to introduce the patient to a healthier lifestyle

✦ Random urine screening for drugs and breath screening for alcohol to monitor abstinence
✦ Family therapy and education to engage and support the family in the recovery process, understand the particular family dynamics, and provide information on chemical dependency as a family disease
✦ Aftercare planning for continued outpatient treatment

Basic medical services are provided on site and in medical specialty services by referral. Following completion of the inpatient phase of treatment, outpatient aftercare (including individual, family, or group psychotherapy or some combination of these) is provided for up to 2 years (Alterman et al. 1991; Chappel 1992; Frances and Franklin 1989; Gallant 1987; Group for the Advancement of Psychiatry 1991; Sternberg 1989; Weiss and Mirin 1989). For some patients, more intensive outpatient care (e.g., day or evening treatment) is required before the patient is ready for the less intensive aftercare phase.

Role of the Psychiatrist

With appropriate training and clinical experience, the psychiatrist is ideally suited to lead the inpatient unit's multidisciplinary treatment team of consulting internists, family physicians or pediatricians, nurses, certified addiction counselors, family therapists, social workers, psychologists, activities therapists, chaplains or pastors, and vocational counselors. The psychiatrist may provide medical management of both the detoxification and continuing intensive treatment in consultation with other physicians as needed.

Specialized inpatient dual-diagnosis treatment programs have recently evolved in response to the increasing recognition of the size and importance of the group of patients with both a substance use disorder and a non–substance-related psychiatric disorder. Most programs strive to integrate traditional psychiatric treatment principles with addiction recovery principles to organize the "two disease concept" and guide effective treatment (Evans and Sullivan 1990; Sternberg 1989; Weiss and Mirin 1989; Wilens 1993). The well-trained psychiatrist is particularly important in providing diagnostic clarification and treatment of both the substance use disorder and the comorbid psychiatric illness. Addiction treatment as previously described is augmented with individual psychotherapy and pharmacotherapy (preferably with drugs that do not have the potential to produce dependence), psychoeducation to discuss the appropriate use of therapeutic medication and the interaction between the addictive and psychiatric illness, and participation in "double trouble" or dual-diagnosis AA and NA meetings. The multidisciplinary team approach, treatment philosophy, goals, and modalities are modeled after those of the inpatient addiction programs. Following the completion of the inpatient phase of treatment, the dual-diagnosis patient enters outpatient care as described above.

In some treatment systems, inpatient detoxification may take place in a separate physical location from the continuing intensive inpatient treatment (e.g., detoxification unit, "scatter beds" in a general hospital). If detoxification is provided in a separate location, special emphasis is placed on motivating the patient for continuing postdetoxification treatment and on preparing the most appropriate treatment plan for the patient. This may involve transition to one of a variety of levels of care, including intensive inpatient, residential, intensive outpatient (e.g., partial hospitalization), or less intensive outpatient care. Outpatient care may be combined with a residential placement (e.g., halfway house, recovery home).

Although most patients remain in inpatient programs anywhere from 1 to several weeks, there are some intensive residential programs of longer duration. Long-term residential treatment of 3–12 months typically serves adolescents (i.e., patients ages 12–18 years). Some adolescents require extended drug-free residential treatment because of the severity of their substance use disorder, their lack of adequate coping skills, the existence of a comorbid psychiatric disorder, or the presence of particularly difficult environmental factors. Treatment is generally based on the 12-step recovery philosophy with regular attendance at self-help meetings. Within a structured disciplined environment, individual, group, and family therapy are provided along with addiction education, year-round school, basic health care, and recreational activities. Depending on the treatment program, the role of the psychiatrist varies from leading a multidisciplinary team to providing consultation on an as-needed basis. Treatment plans, length of stay, and aftercare recommendations are individualized according to the patient's progress in treatment.

Outpatient Settings, Including Private Practice

Consultation, Evaluation, and Intervention

With other health professionals. Psychiatrists are available to provide consult to fellow physicians on individual patients in outpatient as well as inpatient settings. Liaison possibilities also exist in outpatient services (e.g., medical-surgical clinics, group practices, specialized services such as dialysis centers). Some settings have higher rates of substance use disorders than others (e.g., gastroenterology clinics, walk-in clinics that treat minor surgical trauma). The availability and responsiveness of psychiatric consultation increases the access patients with substance use disorders have to appropriate care.

Other mental health professionals turn to psychiatrists for both the pharmacotherapy and the management of patients who are diagnostically or therapeutically challenging. The sensitivity of the consultant to substance use disorders as a mimic or complicator of other psychiatric diagnoses is of special value here. The psychiatrist's willingness to treat difficult and complicated patients is also important. Clinicians in the field of addictive disorders who have limited general mental health training also routinely call on consultants in addiction psychiatry.

In work settings. Institutions and industries have attempted to respond to alcohol and other drug problems in their settings in a variety of ways. Some desire to screen out or fire any employee found to have a substance use problem. Other administrators have supported employee assistance programs (EAPs) wherein an employee who presents with a problem has the opportunity to receive consultation, treatment, or both. Other institutions weigh the value of the employee to the organization before choosing which way to respond.

The EAP model owes its origins in part to the efforts of recovering alcoholic employees who convinced several industries of the value of rehabilitating workers whose alcohol use had been problematic for the company. The success of EAPs has had much to do with promoting addiction treatment. It is unfortunate that many EAPs are organizationally separate from employee health services or the company physician or nurse. Psychiatrists have been associated as consultants or in liaison relationships with the EAPs, but have seldom been directly involved. Only since the EAP model has been expanded to include other employee mental health problems have psychiatrists become more frequently involved.

The EAP model has been applied to hospitals, medical schools, and other health care institutions. In addition, impaired physician programs have been set up by state medical societies throughout the country. Psychiatrists have been active in advocating for the establishment of such programs. They also participate in the assessment, intervention, diagnosis, and treatment of colleagues who have addictive disorders.

In schools.   Schools have also expanded their efforts at curbing substance use and related problems. Initial efforts were directed primarily at early education, with psychiatrists occasionally being invited as guest experts or lecturers. More recently, secondary and high schools have come to embrace a student assistance program model, bringing the benefits of a modified EAP model to the school. Universities face a broader challenge in that part of the student body is of legal drinking age and part is not. They must find a position in a spectrum that ranges from a "dry" campus to one that includes school-sponsored activities during which students age 21 years or older are allowed to drink in moderation. In addition to the need for student assistance services, universities have encountered an increasing number of students in recovery from addictive disorders who would benefit from on-campus support groups and alcohol-free housing. Psychiatric consultants may help responsible administrators develop and run these programs.

To the criminal justice system.   Psychiatrists are also involved in consultation with various components of the criminal justice system. Evaluation and referral to treatment of individuals accused of criminal behavior related to a substance use disorder is a valuable contribution at every stage of the procedure. Evidence of diagnosis and successful initial treatment of these disorders has a significant influence on the sentences imposed for substance-related crimes. Many jurisdictions have screening programs for individuals convicted of driving while impaired or intoxicated to which psychiatrists may provide consultation. This screening and early intervention model could be usefully extended to substance-related domestic violence and other areas.

To families of addicted persons. In addition, psychiatrists are often approached for consultation by family members or significant others of substance-addicted individuals. The intent of the family member to see that the individual receives help is complicated by the impact and meaning of the addiction to the consultee. The psychiatrist may be asked how to approach, intervene with, or even commit the addict. A consultation with a significant other presents opportunities to intervene directly with the addict, as well as to help the significant other with information, support, self-examination, and even direct clinical services.

The Medical Review Officer

As the movement to establish drug-free workplaces gathered momentum during the 1980s, many industrial settings undertook programs of chemical laboratory testing for drugs of abuse. In some cases, this testing was required by law; in others, testing programs were undertaken voluntarily. Current workplace programs may include pre-employment testing, random testing for employees in sensitive positions, testing for all employees, testing after an industrial accident, or testing "for cause" when an employee appears to be under the influence of alcohol or other drugs. For the results of these tests to be interpreted accurately and fairly, review by a physician with appropriate training is required. This physician is called a *medical review officer* (MRO).

The role of the MRO was first defined in 1988 when the Department of Health and Human Services published its guidelines for federal workplace drug testing. These regulations required that all laboratory results be transmitted to a MRO who determines whether or not there are legitimate medical explanations for positive tests (Swotinsky 1992).

The MRO must have a thorough knowledge of pharmacology, laboratory testing, federal regulations, and legal and ethical requirements as well as competence in addiction medicine. He or she is responsible for checking the appropriateness of the testing procedure (including the adequacy of the chain of custody of the specimen) as well as interpreting test results. The MRO is often called on to evaluate an employee who tests positive, and may intervene and refer such employees to the company's EAP or to addiction treatment where indicated.

Several training programs are available for MROs, such as those sponsored by the American College of Occupational and Environmental Medicine and the American Society of Addiction Medicine. Psychiatrists with an interest in addiction have assumed this role for corporations, both on a salaried and consultant basis. With increasing interest in occupational safety and health, and with requirements such as those promulgated by federal agencies (e.g., the Department of Transportation), there will be a growing need for trained MROs. Addiction psychiatrists will play an increasing role in the development of this field.

Specialized Outpatient Addiction Treatment Programs

Outpatient detoxification.   Outpatient detoxification serves as an entry point into the addiction treatment system. It allows for discontinuation of alcohol and other drug use in a safe, medically supervised setting. Pharmacological intervention may or may not be part of the treatment, but the scope of treatment goes beyond simple medical withdrawal.

Outpatient detoxification generally includes assessment of health status, especially whether the patient has any infectious diseases or other complications of substance abuse-dependence. Psychiatric history and mental status examination are also part of the assessment. Psychosocial interventions and referral to AA and other self-help groups are commonly offered. Postdischarge planning and motivation for further treatment are emphasized as critical to long-term recovery. Family involvement is also encouraged.

Outpatient detoxification is appropriately used in a wide variety of cases, except when medical and safety considerations require close medical supervision. The medical role is often limited and of short duration. Hands-on treatment is carried out primarily by nonphysician medical or paramedical personnel.

Treatment goals are usually limited to immediate cessation of substance use and engagement in other ongoing treatment. There is usually limited access to comprehensive medical care at the treatment site. Most medical needs are addressed by referral to other facilities. Patients are educated regarding the nature of addiction and the range of available long-term options and are motivated to enter into long-term treatment. Even for those patients who initially refuse further treatment, repeated cycles of detoxification can serve to decrease alcohol and other drug use and to build motivation for further treatment.

Both pharmacological and nonpharmacological strategies are used to relieve symptoms of withdrawal. Some examples of pharmacological intervention are methadone detoxification, clonidine-assisted detoxification, and buprenorphine detoxification for opiate withdrawal; phenobarbital substitution for sedative-hypnotic (including benzodiazepine) withdrawal; and dopaminergic and serotonergic drugs for cocaine withdrawal, although the latter have produced mixed results.

The psychiatrist can serve as team leader in a multidisciplinary outpatient treatment team. Psychiatrists are in an ideal position to oversee medical detoxification and manage psychiatric comorbidity. As physicians, they can reduce treatment barriers by facilitating communication with other medical colleagues. Their pharmacological expertise ensures quality and integration of treatment and gives confidence to nonmedical members of the treatment team. Psychiatrists are well placed to diagnose and manage confusing behavioral problems arising from substance use, withdrawal, and true psychiatric comorbidity. When necessary, psychiatrists also have the training and authority to initiate involuntary hospitalization.

Intensive outpatient or partial hospitalization programs. The intensive outpatient program model has been increasingly adopted as a lower cost alternative to residential rehabilitation. This model combines individual assessment and treatment with the group spirit and milieu of an intensive inpatient treatment unit, while allowing the patient to live at home. Programs range from a full-day, 7 day-a-week schedule, to half-day or evening programs that are gradually reduced in frequency. Program elements are generally the same as those used in specialized inpatient programs (see section on specialized inpatient programs, above). Both detoxification and continuing treatment may be provided. Some intensive outpatient programs specialize in particular subpopulations of addicted patients, such as adolescents, addicted individuals with significant psychiatric comorbidity, patients with acquired immunodeficiency syndrome, late-stage debilitated alcoholic patients, or addicted individuals with multiple social problems. Emphases on socialization, skill building, activities of daily living, and vocational rehabilitation may complement the treatment of these patients. Lengths of treatment range from several weeks for more intact patients to several months for the chronically and severely ill patients.

Intensive outpatient programs are staffed by interdisciplinary teams similar to those found in inpatient programs. Medical care is usually provided through referral. The psychiatrist may function as the team leader, a team member, or a consultant, depending on the program structure.

For patients to profit from intensive treatment, safe housing and transportation are needed. For some, this may mean living in a community residence or recovery home. Transportation may be a problem in suburban or rural areas, particularly for patients who have lost their driver's licenses because of alcohol or other drug-related infractions. For such patients, special arrangements such as car pools or van service are needed. As is the case with intensive inpatient programs, an aftercare plan consisting of outpatient individual, group, or family therapy or a combination of these therapies in addition to participation in self-help groups follows the intensive treatment phase.

Methadone and other opiate maintenance programs.   Methadone maintenance treatment for opiate addiction was introduced by Dole and Nyswander in 1965. With leadership from the White House Special Action Office for Drug Abuse Prevention and the help of federal grant programs, methadone maintenance treatment (i.e., the prescription of methadone in combination with counseling and rehabilitative services) became widely available in the United States.

Pharmacologically, methadone is a synthetic opioid-agonist, acting primarily at μ-opioid receptors, that maintains a relatively steady blood level for 24–36 hours when given orally. This prevents the rapid fluctuations associated with short-acting narcotics (Dole 1988) and allows the individual on methadone maintenance to function normally in everyday activities. An optimal dosage (blood levels between 150 and 600 ng/ml) prevents withdrawal symptoms, reduces craving, and prevents the high associated with heroin use (Zweben and Payte 1990). Dosages of 60–80 mg daily, up to 100–120 mg daily, are adequate to reduce heroin use and facilitate social rehabilitation while producing only minimal side effects. Higher methadone dosages have been found to result in better treatment outcome than low dosages (20–50 mg daily), and long-term treatment has been found advantageous (Cooper et al. 1983). Despite these findings, in their 1992 nationwide survey of a randomly selected representative sample of methadone clinics, D'Aunno and Vaughn found that practices varied widely, and that about one-quarter of the programs prescribed 60 mg per day or less. The average daily methadone dosage for the majority of programs was 50 mg or less. In addition, half of the programs encouraged maintenance for less than 6 months before movement to drug-free treatment. National experts have expressed concern about the adequacy of these practices (Greenhouse 1992).

Although methadone maintenance treatment has been found to be both effective and cost beneficial (Gerstein and Harwood 1990), several problems have been identified with it. The first of these is that for a methadone maintenance program to be effective, additional services beyond the provision of the methadone are necessary. In a random controlled trial, McLellan et al. (1993) compared the effectiveness of methadone alone, methadone plus counseling, and methadone, counseling, and on-site medical, psychiatric, employment, and family services. They found that the addition of counseling and other services produced a dramatic increase in treatment effectiveness. Even though the provision of these services adds to the cost of methadone maintenance, they are necessary to achieve rehabilitation. A second set of problems derives from the need for daily doses. The provision of take-home methadone doses to alleviate the problem of daily clinic attendance may result in diversion and the creation of a street methadone market, as well as accidental (frequently pediatric) overdose deaths. Also, the selling of methadone in locations adjacent to methadone clinics and the criminal activities associated with such drug diversion have resulted in community dissatisfaction with and resistance to opiate treatment clinics in some neighborhoods. Thus, although for almost 30 years the methadone maintenance model has proven to be a very effective substitution therapy for the opiate-addicted patient, it is not without shortcomings. These shortcomings have led to the stigmatization of methadone treatment in some areas, keeping it from being part of the mainstream health care delivery system.

Problems related to methadone treatment have given impetus to the development of new opiate substitution pharmacotherapies, resulting in the introduction and clinical evaluation of two alternative opiate substitution agents: LAAM and buprenorphine.

LAAM (levo-alpha-acetylmethadol) was formally approved by the Food and Drug Administration in 1993 for use as a maintenance treatment agent for opiate dependence. The opioid effect of LAAM is slower in onset and longer in duration (up to 72 hours) than that of methadone (24 hours). Its extended duration of action allows for three-times-weekly administration. This dosing schedule provides patients more time for employment, educational, and family activities.

In controlled clinical trials, LAAM was found comparable to methadone with respect to reduction of illicit opiate use and treatment retention. The overall results revealed few differences between the two opiate substitution agents in terms of employment, clinic attendance, involvement in illegal activities, and arrests (Blaine et al. 1981). The unique pharmacological characteristics of LAAM and its different mode of clinical delivery are expected to offer an attractive addition to methadone for maintenance treatment.

Buprenorphine is a potent opioid analgesic that possesses both a partial agonist action at the mu and kappa receptors and an antagonist property at the delta receptor. Unlike LAAM, it remains an investigational pharmacotherapy for treatment of opiate addiction, although it is approved in the United States for analgesic use. Buprenorphine induces a low level of opiate physical dependence. Abrupt discontinuation after prolonged buprenorphine treatment results in only a mild morphinelike withdrawal (Jasinski et al. 1978). Several large-scale studies are currently investigating the utility of buprenorphine in maintenance treatment. Available data suggest that the drug may play an important future role in maintenance treatment.

Once stabilized, patients may remain on methadone or LAAM anywhere from 1 year to several years. Methadone and LAAM treatment programs may be freestanding or part of a multimodality addiction program. Staffing may include physicians, nurses, addiction counselors, psychologists, social workers, and vocational counselors. Services offered include physical and mental status evaluation, prescription, dosage evaluation and ongoing management of methadone or LAAM, psychoeducation, addiction counseling, social casework, and a variety of rehabilitative services. Regular breath and urine testing is performed to monitor abstinence from nonopiate drugs of abuse, including alcohol. Medical and psychiatric treatment for comorbidities may be provided on site or by referral. The psychiatrist may be medical director of the program or may function as a staff member or consultant.

With the introduction of newer drugs, maintenance treatment may become more integrated into mainstream medical and psychiatric care, both for helping opiate-addicted individuals and as a useful societal strategy in deterring the spread of HIV. Psychiatrists may play an increasing role in the provision of these maintenance treatments for opiate addiction.

Other specialized addiction outpatient programs. Ambulatory treatment is the most common type of specialized addiction treatment provided in the United States. In the 1991 National Drug and Alcoholism Treatment Unit Survey (NDATUS; Substance Abuse and Mental Health Services Administration 1992a), it was found that about 560,000 of the 809,000 patients receiving care on the survey date were in outpatient facilities, compared with about 8,000 in outpatient detoxification, 42,000 in intensive outpatient treatment (e.g., partial hospitalization), 99,000 in methadone treatment, and the remainder in residential settings. Although some of these clinics identified themselves as "drug free" to distinguish their services from methadone maintenance treatment, most ambulatory programs did prescribe other medications when needed (e.g., disulfiram, antidepressants).

Specialized outpatient programs serve patients entering the treatment system for the first time as well as those moving from a more intensive level of care (e.g., inpatient detoxification, partial hospitalization). These programs tend to be flexible in their hours of operation and frequency of visits. Although initial treatment may involve several sessions per week, the frequency of contact is gradually reduced as recovery proceeds. Patients who run into difficulties or relapse will attend more frequently. Services offered may include

✦ Thorough assessment, including psychosocial history and physical and mental status examination
✦ Psychoeducation about addictive disorders, their effects on individuals and families, the 12-step philosophy, nutrition, HIV infection, and other related subjects
✦ Individual and group addiction counseling
✦ Family therapy
✦ Individual and group counseling for significant others
✦ Behavioral therapies of various types
✦ Vocational evaluation and counseling
✦ Referral to AA, NA, or other self-help groups

✦ Alcohol and other drug testing to monitor continued abstinence
✦ Liaison with EAPs, probation, parole, or other referral sources who may be involved in tracking the patient's progress

Some programs offer psychological testing and psychiatric services on site for patients with serious psychiatric comorbidity, whereas others refer patients to psychiatric outpatient programs for treatment in a coordinated treatment plan. In most facilities, medical, surgical, pediatric, obstetric, and other related services are provided through referral. Special needs (e.g., remedial education, vocational training, financial support) are also usually handled through referral. Some patients attending ambulatory addiction programs reside in halfway houses or specialized community residences. Outpatient programs may specialize in treating specific populations such as women, adolescents, those with HIV infection, or socially disadvantaged or chronically debilitated patients.

The length of treatment in outpatient facilities varies with patient need. A high initial dropout rate is a problem for many facilities. In general, positive outcome correlates with the patient's length of stay in outpatient care (Gerstein and Harwood 1990). It is typical for those who continue to abstain from substance use to remain in treatment for anywhere from several months to 2 years, with a decreasing frequency of contact during that time. Patients who become integrated into strong alcohol- and drug-free support networks, such as self-help programs, continue in those groups after formal outpatient care is completed.

Staffing patterns in outpatient programs depend on the types of services provided, but most programs employ an interdisciplinary team. Addiction counselors characteristically make up a significant proportion of the clinical staff, along with physicians, nurses, psychologists, social workers, rehabilitation counselors, and other professionals. Psychiatrists often assume the role of medical director in outpatient programs. Alternatively, they may be full- or part-time team members or provide services on a consultant basis. In some cases, psychiatrists in private practice provide psychotherapy and pharmacotherapy to ambulatory addiction program patients with comorbid psychiatric disorders in a coordinated treatment plan.

Private practice considerations. The psychiatrist in private practice will be called on for consultation-liaison and intervention services as described in the section "Consultation, Evaluation, and Intervention," above. In some cases, a psychoactive substance use disorder may be the presenting problem. The psychiatrist is in the unique, advantageous position of being able to establish the patient's diagnosis, provide medical detoxification, institute individual psychotherapeutic and pharmacological treatment, and work in the context of group, network, or other recovery-oriented social therapies.

The efficacy of detoxification in the private practice setting can be improved when augmented by psychotherapy (Otto et al. 1993). A range of psychotherapeutic approaches can be applied effectively to addiction treatment (Kaufman and Reoux 1988; Woody et al. 1987; Zimberg et al. 1985), including psychodynamic (Kaufman 1992; Khantzian 1986) and cognitive-behavior approaches (Beck et al. 1993). Traditional concepts of therapeutic structure have also been modified to serve addicted patients effectively (e.g., groups [Khantzian et al. 1992; Vannicelli 1992], networks [Galanter 1993]). Pharmacological therapies, such as disulfiram (Gorelick 1983) and naltrexone (Volpicelli et al. 1992), are effective agents in the practitioner's armamentarium. Recovery-oriented support systems are often provided by referral of both patients and family members to self-help fellowships as a treatment adjunct. Comorbid psychiatric illness can be treated along with the addictive disorder. Regular chemical testing for alcohol or other drugs often accompanies office treatment.

Substance use disorders do not always present themselves as the primary problem. The patient may seek psychiatric treatment for depression, anxiety, or behavioral problems. Because of the high prevalence of substance use disorders in patients with other psychiatric disorders, the individual practitioner should include examination for addictive illness as part of the standard evaluation of all patients. When a substance use disorder—whether identified initially or discovered in the course of treatment of another psychiatric disorder—is addressed directly, a successful outcome often follows (McLellan et al. 1987).

Private psychiatric practice is also a common and useful setting for ongoing follow-up care after a patient has been discharged from inpatient care, an intensive outpatient-partial hospitalization program, or a residential facility. Recovery from addiction matures over time and may require a spectrum of pharmacological, psychotherapeutic, and interpersonal therapies.

Outpatient Psychiatric Treatment Programs

Traditional psychiatric outpatient clinics usually do not draw patients who present with a chief complaint of substance use disorders. However, as with the evaluation of psychiatric inpatients, every initial workup should include screening for these disorders. When measured as part of a research study, the rates of substance abuse–dependence among both adolescent and adult psychiatric clinic outpatients are found to be consistently higher than believed by the clinic staff. When substance use continues during psychiatric treatment, improvement rates are low and rates of hospitalization are high (Ridgeley et al. 1989). Former inpatients also have a higher risk of rehospitalization if they persist in substance use. Some patients with serious Axis I disorders and comorbid substance use disorders do better with brief supportive visits oriented around pharmacological management than with confrontational techniques or interactive groups (Gottheil and Warren 1982). It is therefore important in treating these patients to integrate addictive disorder treatment with traditional outpatient psychiatric care. Other patients may profit from a joint treatment plan that includes psychiatric and substance use treatment delivered in a coordinated manner at two different outpatient settings. Still others require a specialized dual-diagnosis outpatient program for maximum benefit. In each of these models, participation of the appropriately trained psychiatrist is of critical importance.

Nicotine Dependence Treatment

A variety of approaches to treatment of nicotine dependence have been developed since the 1960s. Most have been outpatient methods designed for general medical practice or specialized smoking-cessation clinics (Preventive Services Task Force 1989). More recently, both in- and outpatient programs for treatment of alcohol and other drug abuse–dependence have begun to offer concurrent treatment for nicotine dependence (Karan 1993).

Among outpatient approaches, brief physician intervention alone has been found to have some positive effect (Preventive Services Task Force 1989). Motivational counseling may be combined with nicotine replacement and gradual detoxification, with either transdermal nicotine patches or nicotine polacrilex chewing gum being used. Other pharmacological approaches to nicotine withdrawal treatment have been attempted (e.g., clonidine detoxification) as have hypnosis and acupuncture. Behavioral treatment modalities include aversion, relaxation training, and nicotine fading (gradual cessation of smoking), among other individual and group approaches. Many programs combine several modalities with continuing supportive contact (Preventive Services Task Force 1989).

In addition, a variety of self-help manuals and self-help groups, most notably Smokers Anonymous, are available to aid in the treatment of nicotine dependence.

Psychiatrists may use any of the above techniques in private practice, outpatient settings, or inpatient psychiatric units, as well as in programs for the treatment of substance use disorders. The growing movement to make hospitals smoke free, combined with an increasing concern about the long-term health effects of tobacco use, have encouraged psychiatrists to become involved in nicotine dependence treatment.

Social Setting Detoxification

The terms *social setting detox, sobering-up station,* and *subacute detoxification center* are used in various parts of the country to describe facilities designed to allow alcohol-intoxicated individuals or individuals in mild alcohol withdrawal to sober up in a safe and medically supervised setting. Many states decriminalized public intoxication during the 1970s. This provided impetus for the establishment of such facilities as replacements for the so-called drunk tanks in local jails, in which individuals who were intoxicated in public were incarcerated to "sleep it off." These cells were often unsanitary and dangerous. Little or no medical screening or supervision was provided and such complications as seizures, hallucinations, and severe withdrawal states were common. In addition, head injuries, diabetic coma, suicidal depression, and other life-threatening conditions were sometimes overlooked with the assumption that the individual was "just drunk" (Institute of Medicine 1990).

According to the Institute of Medicine (1990), the goals of the social setting detoxification unit include

✦ Screening for illness, injury, suicidal intent, or severe withdrawal
✦ Immediate referral for medical care (often by written contract with a general hospital emergency service) when needed
✦ Provision of a safe clean and supervised environment in which to recover from intoxication
✦ Provision of at least an initial assessment of the client's alcohol abuse-dependence and associated problems
✦ Provision of basic personal care, a shower, clean clothing, and nutrition
✦ Provision of psychoeducation and motivational counseling
✦ Preparation of a plan for continued treatment after sobriety is attained

Social setting detoxes may be freestanding or organized as part of a larger, multicomponent program. Staffing usually includes at least one registered nurse, specially trained technicians, and possibly alcoholism counselors. A medical director or consultant may set medical policy and advise the staff. In some programs, a medical director makes regular visits. This role may be filled by a psychiatrist.

Components of care include a general assessment for bodily injury or illness, the taking of vital signs, a breath test to screen for blood alcohol level, and as much initial history as the patient can provide, including questions about the substances ingested and the patient's mood and suicidal thoughts. The patient is given a shower if indicated and observed closely with frequent vital signs taken. As he or she recovers, further assessment, counseling, and aftercare planning are provided. The average length of stay is 2–4 days, although some centers may retain patients for longer periods, particularly if they are awaiting housing or treatment program placement.

Patients may be brought to the unit by police or others acquainted with the program's mission. Many centers have vans that can respond to requests to pick up intoxicated individuals.

The main strength of social setting detoxification programs is that they allow safe and cost-effective detoxification, reserving inpatient hospital detoxification for individuals with more severe or complicated withdrawals. With good initial screening, only a small percentage of patients require subsequent hospital admission. Pressures on such facilities include crowding and the need to keep stays short to accommodate others in need of services, even when the staff feel that a particular patient might respond to motivational counseling if more time were available. Another serious problem for these facilities, which were designed to serve individuals intoxicated by alcohol, is that many drug-intoxicated individuals as well as mentally ill individuals who abuse alcohol also apply to use these services. Policies vary on how such cases are handled, but they present an ongoing challenge.

Community Residences

The term *community residence* is used here to describe a range of facilities generally providing transitional residential services to individuals who have completed some part of their addiction treatment and require the social structure and support of a group living environment during the early phase of recovery. Residents of these facilities may be referred from detoxification or intensive inpatient treatment programs, but may also come from jails, prisons, outpatient programs, or psychiatric facilities.

Both the names given to these programs and their therapeutic organization vary greatly across the United States. *Halfway houses, quarterway houses, domiciliaries, recovery homes,* and *community residences* are all terms in current use. Some of these programs have a resident manager as the only salaried staff. Others are staffed by addiction treatment professionals who conduct ongoing treatment and vocational rehabilitation activities for residents. In the majority of programs, residents carry out most of the basic duties needed to run the facility: governance, meal planning, cooking, cleaning, maintenance, and so on. Addiction treatment and medical care are often provided by local outpatient programs. Self-help meetings may be held in the facility or residents may attend community self-help meetings. An emphasis is placed on maintaining abstinence, working or participating in vocational rehabilitation, developing social skills, and becoming integrated within a supportive alcohol- and drug-free social network. The length of stay ranges from 3 months to 18 months or more, depending on the program type. In addition, facilities may specialize in helping residents with concurrent psychiatric illnesses or adolescents or adults involved with the criminal justice system.

Many insurance policies do not cover care in such facilities (Institute of Medicine 1990). Major funding for these facilities comes from government grants, resident payments (those who are employed or receive public assistance pay a weekly contribution), and charitable donations. Staffing of community residences varies from a sole resident manager (often a trained addiction counselor) to a full staff including social workers, psychologists, counselors, nurses, vocational rehabilitation specialists, and pastoral counselors. Psychiatrists may play varying roles in community residences. They may participate in the original development of the program, provide staff education and consultation, and provide addiction and other psychiatric treatment to residents on an outpatient basis.

Recently, community residences for pregnant and postpartum women (and their children), or for women with small children, have been established in several states. These women's programs are being developed to meet a particularly pressing societal problem: the lack of adequate child care is frequently an insurmountable barrier to addicted mothers of young children, frustrating their access to needed residential treatment. These women are often single parents who lack family or other resources to support their efforts at recovery (Blume, in press). In addition, women who are pregnant are often excluded from residential addiction treatment facilities, even from hospital-based detoxification programs. For example, in a survey of 78 alcohol and drug treatment programs located in New York City, Chavkin (1990) found that 54% refused to accept pregnant women.

However, aided by the 1984 legislative requirement that 5% of the federal alcohol-drug block grant be set aside for women's services, model programs began to be established. Later on, additional direct grants to develop programs for pregnant women were offered by the Alcohol, Drug Abuse and Mental Health Administration (now the Substance Abuse and Mental Health Services Administration). In 1988, the women's set-aside was increased to 10%. The programs for women and children developed in response to these initiatives are not all residential in nature. However, they have in common the provision of a spectrum of services, including coordinated medical, obstetric, pediatric, psychiatric, and addiction treatment, as well as vocational and parenting training for the participating women and services for their children.

Psychiatrists have an important role as providers of treatment to the women and children in these specialized programs, in addition to serving as consultants to the program staff. Women with addictive disorders often have been victims of physical and sexual abuse (Blume 1991). Helping them deal with these issues is a major part of the challenge of women's addiction programs. The psychiatrist is often an indispensable member of the clinical team engaged in this effort.

Therapeutic Communities

Synanon, founded in 1958, was the first of a series of specialized residential programs known as *therapeutic communities.* In its original design, Synanon was not so much aimed at rehabilitation as at the provision of an alternate and separate lifestyle. Its goals were to understand the addicted individual: provide him or her with basic supplies, such as food, clothing, and shelter, and help him or her to find a satisfying role in Synanon's drug-free community (Cherkas 1965).

In the mid-1960s, Daytop Lodge emerged as a new therapeutic community for addicted individuals. Its program emphasized rehabilitation, with the goal of reintegrating the recovering resident into mainstream society. Its success provided the prototype for therapeutic communities and led to their proliferation (O'Brien and Biase 1992). During the ensuing 30 years, therapeutic communities continued to evolve, with the therapeutic community model being applied to settings in the criminal justice system as well as community-based facilities. The goals of contemporary therapeutic communities include changes in lifestyle, abstinence from psychoactive substance use, elimination of antisocial activity, development of employability, and fostering of prosocial attitudes and values (De Leon and Rosenthal 1989).

Therapeutic communities are based on social learning models. Although they stress community, they also emphasize the personal responsibility and accountability of each resident. All activities performed within the community are seen as having rehabilitative value, including work assignments. Each resident, at the beginning of his or her stay, pays his or her "dues" by doing the most basic of chores, such as mopping the floor. As residents progress to higher levels of functioning and status, through both time and participation in the community, they serve as models for the other residents. This "promotability" is perhaps best reflected in the fact that former residents have often remained as staff. Treatment tends to be long-term, with stays of 1–2 years not unusual.

Group methods employed in therapeutic communities include encounters, probes, and marathons (De Leon and Rosenthal 1989). Medical and psychiatric services for therapeutic community residents with comorbid illnesses are usually provided by referral. Because confrontational methods of treatment may be counterproductive or harmful for some addicted individuals, most therapeutic communities have a policy of excluding applicants with serious psychiatric comorbidity. However, some therapeutic communities have recently begun to adapt their programs to accommodate such patients (Carroll 1991).

Staffing usually relies heavily on addiction counselors, many of whom are program "graduates" trained by the therapeutic community. Addiction professionals may also be involved as staff members. Psychiatrists may play a role in developing the program and may provide staff education and consultation. In addition, they may provide diagnosis and treatment to residents in need of these services.

Programs in the Criminal Justice System

On any one day in 1987, nearly 3.7 million adult Americans were under the supervision of the criminal justice system, a number representing almost 2% of the adult population. Although the vast majority of these individuals were on probation (about 2.24 million) or parole (360,000), the remainder were incarcerated in prisons or jails, as were about 50,000 juvenile offenders (Gerstein and Harwood 1990).

Rates of substance use disorders in the incarcerated population are high. As described under "Epidemiology" in Chapter 1, the Epidemiologic Catchment Area (ECA) Study (Regier et al. 1990) documented high rates of substance use disorders among incarcerated populations (72% lifetime prevalence, with alcohol abuse-dependence in 56.2% and other drug abuse-dependence in 53.7%). These rates are in agreement with earlier surveys of substance use histories among prisoners (Frohling 1989; Leukefeld and Tims 1992).

Several models of alcohol and other drug treatment programs have been developed within the criminal justice system. These include pretrial diversion to community-based facilities and the use of treatment as an adjunct to probation or parole. Probationers or parolees may either be referred to community-based treatment as a condition of probation or parole, or, in some states, committed involuntarily to residential programs. The best example of programs providing assessment, referral, and follow-up for diversion or probation-supervised patients is Treatment Alternatives to Street Crime (TASC). Begun with federal assistance in 1972, the TASC network of 180 programs in 29 states and territories is now state funded (National Consortium of Treatment Alternatives to Street Crime Programs 1993). TASC referral is a frequent point of entry into the addiction treatment system.

In addition, both prisons and jails have recognized the need for programs of their own for inmates with serious alcohol and drug problems. However, despite the known high prevalence of substance use disorders among inmates, the development of treatment programs within these facilities has been slow and the quality of programs has been uneven. A 1979 survey of prisons (Tims 1981) found that about 4% of the incarcerated population were involved in 160 prison-based programs, about a third of which were based on a therapeutic community model. By 1987, an estimated 11% of prisoners were in such programs (Chaiken and Johnson 1988). This number, although an improvement, still falls far short of the need. A current snapshot of the national situation was presented in a recent National Institute on Drug Abuse (NIDA) monograph, as follows:

> Forty-four states allow Narcotics Anonymous (NA), Cocaine Anonymous (CA), or Alcoholics Anonymous (AA) self-help group meetings once or twice a week; 44 states have some form of short-term (35 to 50 hours) drug education programming; 31 states have some form of individual counseling available for drug users in which a counselor or therapist meets with an individual inmate occasionally during the week; 36 states have group counseling in which small groups of inmates meet once or twice weekly with a therapist; and 30 states have some type of intensive residential program, often based on the therapeutic community model. Most optimistically, less than 20% of identified drug-using offenders are believed to be served by these programs. (Leukefeld and Tims 1992, p. 12)

The most common treatment model in use is group counseling, alone or combined with 12-step group attendance. Less common is the milieu therapy approach in which program participants live together isolated from the rest of the prison population. In this setting they are offered individual and group counseling by a staff of social workers, psychologists, and specially trained corrections officers (Leukefeld and Tims 1992). In contrast, prison therapeutic communities follow the more intensely interactive model of community-based therapeutic communities. Evaluations of prison-based therapeutic communities have demonstrated important decreases in re-arrest rates after release (Gerstein and Harwood 1990).

In two recent studies, the General Accounting Office (GAO; 1991a, 1991b) assessed the need for programs and their availability in federal and state prisons. These studies noted that the first Public Health Service facilities for drug treatment within the federal prison system were established in the 1930s at maximum security prisons in Lexington, Kentucky, and Forth Worth, Texas. Despite this history, current federal prison addiction treatment programs were found to be inadequate. Among an inmate population of approximately 62,000, the Federal Bureau of Prisons estimated that about 44%—or 27,000—inmates have moderate to severe substance abuse or dependence. However, the GAO found that only 364 inmates were receiving intensive treatment, representing only half the available capacity.

In the GAO's study of state prison systems (General Accounting Office 1991b), conducted in 1990 and 1991, only approximately 20% of those in need of treatment were receiving it. Counseling and residential treatment were the modalities most often employed (Swanson et al. 1993).

Less has been written about jail-based programs than prison-based programs. Because jails have a more transient population, the long-term therapeutic community approach is not feasible. However, jails have been effectively adapted for residential treatment of alcoholic patients jailed after being convicted for driving while intoxicated (usually following multiple convictions) or for probation or parole violators wishing to avoid a return to prison. At Riker's Island jail in New York City, opiate-dependent inmates charged with misdemeanors are allowed to participate in the jail's large methadone maintenance treatment program as an alternative to rapid detoxification; this participation is combined with referral for postjail methadone treatment (Magura et al. 1993).

Goals of a jail- or prison-based addiction treatment program include gaining the interest and motivation of the inmate-patients, educating them about addiction, changing their attitudes toward reintegration into society, initiating drug-free or methadone treatment and connections to self-help programs, motivating inmates for aftercare, and improving inmates' postincarceration adjustment. Abstinence and avoidance of criminal recidivism are the ultimate postrelease goals.

Elements necessary for a successful program were listed in the 1990 Institute of Medicine study on the treatment of drug problems as follows (Gerstein and Harwood 1990, p. 177):

✦ A competent and committed staff
✦ Adequate administrative and material support by correctional authorities
✦ Separation from the general prison population
✦ Incorporation of self-help principles and ex-offender aid
✦ Comprehensive, intensive therapy aimed at the entire lifestyle of a patient and not just the substance abuse aspects
✦ Continuity of care into the parole period—an absolutely essential element

To this list might be added support by the larger community. Psychiatrists working within jail or prison settings may fulfill a variety of roles. They may help organize and establish addiction treatment programs and their policies, screen potential staff members, consult with staff, and supervise clinical activities. They may also provide screening and consultation for program participants. At times the program psychiatrist may also treat and follow up patients within the program (Morton 1993).

The Current Addiction Treatment System

Determining the level of societal need for each of the types and settings of addiction treatment described above has been a difficult problem. In the 1992 National Drug Control Strategy issued by the White House's Office of National Drug Control Policy, it was estimated that there are approximately 2.77 million Americans who need and could benefit from drug abuse-dependence treatment (exclusive of treatment for alcohol and tobacco abuse-dependence). The authors of the report further estimated that, as of 1992, the treatment system provided 599,000 treatment "slots" able to serve approximately 1.7 million Americans each year. Although alcohol abuse-dependence is more prevalent than other drug abuse-dependence, an accepted methodology for assessing the need for alcoholism treatment has not been developed. Current methods rely on the observed level of treatment utilization or demand, to which are added adjustments for demographic factors and various indices of health problems (Institute of Medicine 1990).

Surveys of the current national treatment system have been conducted by NIDA since 1974, and by NIDA jointly with National Institute on Alcohol Abuse and Alcoholism since 1979. In 1992, responsibility for the survey, entitled the National Drug and Alcoholism Treatment Unit Survey (NDATUS), was taken over by the Office of Applied Studies of the Substance Abuse and Mental Health Services Administration (SAMHSA). NDATUS is a periodic point prevalence survey of all known alcohol and drug prevention and treatment programs. The last fully reported survey was conducted on September 30, 1991, with the help of the State Alcohol and Drug Abuse Agencies. Data from 11,277 prevention and treatment units, which represented 81% of all identified programs, were collected.

The NDATUS methodology has several limitations. For example, some multiservice programs are reported as a single unit, whereas others are reported as several units. In addition, the data are not adjusted statistically for nonresponding units. Nevertheless, the NDATUS represents the best available cross-sectional description of the current specialty addiction treatment system.

Highlights of the NDATUS findings for 1991 (Substance Abuse and Mental Health Services Administration 1992a) compared, where possible, with preliminary 1992 NDATUS data (Substance Abuse and Mental Health Services Administration 1992b) and 1989 NDATUS data (National Institute of Drug Abuse and National Institute on Alcohol Abuse and Alcoholism 1990) are shown in Table 2–1. More than 800,000 patients were reported to be in addiction treatment on September 30, 1991, by 9,057 treatment units. The vast majority of these units offered both alcohol and other drug dependence treatment. Methadone treatment was offered in 604 of these units, often in conjunction with other alcohol and drug treatment services. According to the survey data, a total treatment capacity (counting all types of treatment) of 1,002,385 "slots" were available on the day of the survey in reporting units. Eighty-seven percent of the system's treatment capacity was in ambulatory care, with 10.9% in residential services and only 1.8% in inpatient detoxification.

In Table 2–2, utilization rates for those programs reporting both patient census and treatment capacity on the day of the survey are shown. Utilization rates were highest in longer term residential units (84.5%) and outpatient treatment (82.6%). Freestanding residential detoxification programs (primarily social setting detoxes) had a 75.7% utilization rate, whereas the utilization rate for hospital detoxification units was only 57.6%. Other rates were hospital inpatient rehabilitation, 63.3%; short-term residential (30 days or less), 74.8%; and intensive outpatient and outpatient detoxification, 69.8% and 66.3%, respectively. Preliminary 1992 data (Substance

Table 2–1. Treatment units and patients from the 1991 National Drug and Alcoholism Treatment Unit Survey (NDATUS) (compared with 1989 data and preliminary 1992 data where available)

	1992	1991	1989
Treatment units			
Total number of reporting treatment units (including methadone)	9,483	9,057	7,759
Number of methadone treatment units	659	604	—[a]
Number (%) of alcohol-only treatment units	1,186 (12.5%)	984 (10.9%)	—[a]
Number (%) of drug-only treatment units	978 (10.3%)	896 (9.9%)	—[a]
Number (%) of combined treatment units	7,319 (77.2%)	7,177 (79.2%)	—[a]
Patients			
Total patients in treatment on 9/30/91	794,755	811,819	734,955
Alcoholism patients (%)	290,040 (36.5%)	365,147 (45.0%)	383,525 (52%)
Drug abuse patients (%)	214,736 (27%)	237,008 (29.2%)	351,430 (48%)
Patients with both problems (%)	289,979 (36.5%)	209,664 (25.8%)	—[a]

[a]No data provided.
Sources. National Institute on Drug Abuse and National Institute on Alcohol Abuse and Alcoholism 1990; Office of Applied Studies, Substance Abuse and Mental Health Services Administration 1992a, 1992b.

Abuse and Mental Health Services Administration 1992b) are shown in the table for comparison. In the NDATUS, it is documented that 99,111 patients were in methadone treatment on September 30, 1991. Among all methadone programs reporting both census and treatment capacity, 85.7% of that capacity was in use. It is interesting that utilization rates varied with unit ownership. The rate was lowest in private, for-profit units (70%) as compared with federal government units (74.7%), tribal government units (76.7%), private nonprofit units (82.4%), and state and local government units (85.7%). Unit ownership and numbers of patients in treatment are shown in Table 2–3 for 1991 and 1989.

Critics of NDATUS have identified several additional shortcomings of the survey. The 1990 Institute of Medicine study pointed out that the broad categories of treatment in the 1989 NDATUS survey (National Institute on

Table 2–2. Number of patients in treatment by type of care and utilization of treatment capacity, September 30, 1991 (compared with preliminary 1992 data where available)

	Patients		**Utilization rate (%)**[a]	
	1991	**1992**	**1991**	**1992**
Detoxification				
Inpatient, hospital based	5,198	9,017	57.6	46.7
Freestanding, residential	6,256	8,268	75.7	80.9
Rehabilitation/residential				
Inpatient, hospital based	9,183	14,501	63.3	64.4
Short-term (30 days or less)	17,294	23,114	74.8	76.5
Long-term (more than 30 days)	60,418	71,469	84.5	82.0
Outpatient treatment				
Outpatient detoxification	7,912	11,928	66.3	70.8
Intensive outpatient treatment	42,032	60,246	69.8	70.4
Other outpatient (including 99,111 in methadone treatment)	661,031	799,934	82.6	83.0
Total	809,324	998,477	81.1	81.4

[a]Numbers only for units reporting both census and treatment capacity.
Sources. Substance Abuse and Mental Health Services Administration 1992a, 1992b.

Table 2–3. Ownership of treatment units and number of patients in treatment from the 1989 and 1991 National Drug and Alcoholism Treatment Unit Surveys (NDATUS) (compared with preliminary 1992 data)

Ownership	No. treatment units			No. patients		
	1992	**1991**	**1989**	**9/30/92**	**9/30/91**	**9/30/89**
Private, for profit	1,765	1,675	1,258	121,251	124,952	91,632
Private, nonprofit	5,842	5,744	4,958	448,312	460,970	431,576
State and local government	1,345	1,341	1,236	173,174	194,826	171,907
Federal government	243	211	190	26,810	25,920	23,851
Tribal government	66	63	N/A	2,072	3,081	N/A

Sources. National Institute on Drug Abuse and National Institute on Alcohol Abuse and Alcoholism 1990; Office of Applied Studies, Substance Abuse and Mental Health Services Administration 1992a, 1992b.

Drug Abuse and National Institute on Alcohol Abuse and Alcoholism 1990) were difficult to interpret because the survey designers lumped several types of care together. In the 1991 NDATUS report (Substance Abuse and Mental Health Services Administration 1992a), longer and shorter term residential care, ambulatory detoxification, and intensive outpatient were separated out from other outpatient treatment for the first time. However, the "other" outpatient category still combined different types and intensities of care. Further criticism has been focused on the value of NDATUS as an accurate snapshot of the nation's addiction treatment capacity given that it completely omits individuals involved in self-help, those receiving care in the private practices of general medical and mental health professionals, and those in treatment in facilities not identified as addiction treatment programs (e.g., community mental health centers, psychiatric units) (Schlesinger and Dorwart 1992). Thus, the data provided in NDATUS represent an underestimation of the actual national treatment capacity and the numbers of persons actually receiving services.

Data derived from the ECA Study (Regier et al. 1990) verified the observation that many more adults with substance use disorders receive help outside of specialty alcohol and drug treatment programs than within them (Narrow et al. 1993). The study defined *services* very broadly to include self-help; help from a friend or relative, clergyperson, or social agency; and services from a medical, psychiatric, or alcohol or drug treatment facility. The ECA analysis found that only 11% of individuals with substance use disorders who received help during a 1-year period used alcohol or drug treatment clinics (4.7% Veterans Administration clinics, 6.3% other clinics), representing only 7.7% of all outpatient service visits for that year. Self-help was used by 7.9% of the alcohol- or drug-affected individuals who received some form of help, accounting for 20.6% of visits. A far greater percentage were seen by mental health professionals in private practice (16%), in mental health clinics (10.1%), or in health plan settings (7.5%). As many outpatient visits were made to physicians in general medical settings as were made to alcohol or drug treatment programs. These trends were particularly evident for individuals with comorbid non–substance-related mental disorders. A comparison of ECA data on service utilization with data from other studies has revealed a general congruence (Manderscheid et al. 1993), indicating that the picture offered by the ECA is probably accurate.

Examining the treatment received by individuals suffering from addictive disorders from this wider perspective, several questions arise. First of all, it is not possible to estimate how much of the utilization of non–addiction-specific sources of help is a result of the shortage or maldistribution of alcohol and other drug treatment programs. Presumably, however, this is an important contributing factor. Similarly, the proportion of patients who had addiction-specific care theoretically available to them but who were shunted to other sources of help because they lacked appropriate insurance coverage or because of other economic barriers cannot be judged from current data. In addition, the ECA Study does not differentiate in its description of sources of help in what is called the *voluntary support network* (e.g., clergy, family, social services agencies) those providers that have staff trained or credentialed to provide addiction-specific care from those providers who lack such staff. Thus the adequacy, or even the specificity, of current care cannot be estimated.

Second, it is evident that a significant number of addicted patients receive care in general medical settings. Considering the findings of underdiagnosis and failure to intervene when these patients interact with the health care system (see "Programs in General Medical Settings," above), the ECA data document an extensive but probably largely missed opportunity for appropriate intervention. The data also suggest an important need for education and training of primary care personnel. Although some of the patients who received their care in the general health system were no doubt treated by nonpsychiatrist addiction-treatment professionals in primary care settings, the vast majority were not. It is this larger number of health care providers who urgently need better training in addictive disorders. In developing such training, a realistic goal must be set. It would seem reasonable to expect that most of these professionals could be trained to provide diagnosis and referral services to addicted patients. However, what is a reasonable expectation for the provision of addiction treatment itself in primary care settings? This question deserves careful study.

Summary

The service system (in its broadest definition) currently used by individuals with substance use disorders consists of a combination of formal and informal resources in the general health, mental health, self-help, and social service sectors in addition to the specialty addiction treatment system.

References

Alterman AI, O'Brien CP, McLellan AT: Differential therapeutics for substance abuse, in Clinical Textbook of Addictive Disorders. Edited by Frances RJ, Miller SI. New York, Guilford Press, 1991, pp 369–390

American Society of Addiction Medicine: Patient Placement Criteria for the Treatment of Psychoactive Substance Use Disorders. Washington, DC, American Society of Addiction Medicine, 1991

Beck AT, Wright FD, Newman CF, et al: Cognitive Therapy of Substance Abuse. New York, Guilford Press, 1993

Beresford TP, Low D, Hall RC, et al: Alcoholism in the general hospital. Psychiatric Medicine 2:139–148, 1984

Blaine JD, Thomas DB, Barnett G, et al: Levo-alpha acetylmethadol (LAAM): clinical utility and pharmaceutical development, in Substance Abuse: Clinical Involvement and Perspectives. Edited by Lowinson JH, Ruiz P. Baltimore, Williams & Wilkins, 1981, pp 360–388

Blume SB: Psychotherapy in the Treatment of Alcoholism, in Psychiatry Update: The American Psychiatric Association Annual Review, Vol 3. Edited by Grinspoon L. Washington, DC, American Psychiatric Press, 1984, pp 338–345

Blume SB: Sexuality and stigma: the alcoholic women. Alcohol Health Research World 15(2):139–146, 1991

Blume SB: Women and alcohol: issues in social policy, in Gender and Alcohol. Edited by Wilsnack RW, Wilsnack SC. New Brunswick, NJ, Rutgers Center of Alcohol Studies (in press)

Buchsbaum DG, Buchanan RG, Centor RM, et al: Screening for alcohol abuse using CAGE scores and likelihood ratios. Ann Intern Med 115:744–777, 1991

Bunt G, Galanter M, Lifschutz H, et al: Cocaine/"crack" dependence in psychiatric in-patients. Am J Psychiatry 147:1542–1546, 1990

Burton RW, Lyons JS, Doucas M, et al: Psychiatric consultations for psychoactive substance abuse disorders in the general hospital. Gen Hosp Psychiatry 13:83–87, 1991

Carroll JFX: Mental health problems of TC residents and their implications for treatment. Paper presented at the XIV World Conference of Therapeutic Communities, "Drugs and Society to the Year 2000," Montreal, Canada, September 1991

Chaiken MR, Johnson BD: Issues and Practices: Characteristics of Different Types of Drug Involved Offenders. National Institute of Justice Research in Brief, Washington, DC, National Institute of Justice, 1988

Chang G, Astrachan BM: The emergency department surveillance of alcohol intoxication after motor vehicle accidents. JAMA 260:2533–2536, 1988

Chappel JN: Effective use of Alcoholics Anonymous and Narcotics Anonymous in treating patients. Psychiatric Annals 22:409–418, 1992

Chavkin W: Drug addiction and pregnancy, policy crossroads. Am J Public Health 80:483–486, 1990

Cherkas MS: Synanon foundation: a radical approach to the problem of addiction. Am J Psychiatry 121:1065–1069, 1965

Cleary PD, Miller M, Bush BT, et al: Prevalence and recognition of alcohol abuse in a primary care population. Am J Med 85:466–471, 1988

Cooper JR, Altman F, Brown BS, et al. (eds): Research on Treatment of Narcotic Addiction: State of the Art. (DHHS Publ No ADM-83-1281). Rockville, MD, National Institute on Drug Abuse, 1983

Crumley F: Substance abuse and adolescent suicidal behavior. JAMA 263:3051–3056, 1990

D'Aunno T, Vaughn TE: Variations in methadone treatment practices. JAMA 267:253–258, 1992

De Leon G, Rosenthal MS: Treatment in residential therapeutic communities, in Treatments of Psychiatric Disorders: A Task Force Report of the American Psychiatric Association, Vol 2. Washington, DC, American Psychiatric Association, 1989, pp 1379–1396

Dole VP: Implications of methadone maintenance for theories of narcotic addiction. JAMA 260:3025–3029, 1988

Dole VP, Nyswander M: A medical treatment for diacetylmorphine [DIACETYL] (heroin) addiction: a clinical trial with methadone hydrochlorides. JAMA 193:80–84, 1965

Evans K, Sullivan JM (eds): Dual Diagnosis: Counseling the Mentally Ill Substance Abuser. New York, Guilford Press, 1990

Ewing JA: Detecting alcoholism: the CAGE questionnaire. JAMA 252:1905–1907, 1984.

Frances RJ, Franklin JE: Concise Guide to Treatment of Alcoholism and Addictions. Washington, DC, American Psychiatric Press, 1989

Frances RJ, Miller SI: Addiction treatment: the widening scope, in Clinical Textbook of Addictive Disorders. Edited by Frances RJ, Miller SI. New York, Guilford Press, 1991, pp 3–22

Frohling R: Promising Approaches to Drug Treatment in Correctional Settings. Criminal Justice Paper No 7. Denver, CO, National Conference of State Legislatures, 1989

Galanter M: Network therapy for addiction. Am J Psychiatry 150:28–36, 1993

Galanter M, Castenada R, Ferman J: Substance abuse among psychiatric patients. Am J Drug Alcohol Abuse 14:211–235, 1988

Gallant DM (ed): Alcoholism: A Guide to Diagnosis, Intervention, and Treatment. New York, WW Norton, 1987

General Accounting Office: Drug Treatment: Despite New Strategy Few Federal Inmates Receive Treatment (Publ GAO/HRD 91-166). Washington, DC, General Accounting Office, 1991a

General Accounting Office: Drug Treatment: State Prisons Face Challenges in Providing Services (Publ GAO/HRD 91-128). Washington, DC, General Accounting Office, 1991b

Gentilello L: Major injury as a unique opportunity to initiate treatment in the alcoholic. Am J Surg 156:558–561, 1989

Gerstein DR, Harwood HJ (eds): Treating Drug Problems, Vol 1. Washington, DC, National Academy Press, 1990

Gorelick DA: Pharmacotherapy of alcohol and drug abuse. Psychiatric Annals 13:71–79, 1983

Gottheil E, Warren H: Alcoholism and Schizophrenia, in Encyclopedic Handbook of Alcoholism. Edited by Pattison EM, Kaufman E. New York, Gardner Press, 1982, pp 636–646

Greenhouse CM. Study find methadone treatment practices vary widely in effectiveness. NIDA Notes 7:1–5, 1992

Group for the Advancement of Psychiatry, Committee on Alcoholism and the Addictions: Substance abuse disorders: a psychiatric priority. Am J Psychiatry 148:1291–1300, 1991

Institute of Medicine: Broadening the Base of Treatment for Alcohol Problems. Washington, DC, American Psychiatric Press, 1990

Jasinski DR, Pevnick JS, Griffith JD: Human pharmacology and abuse potential of the analgesic buprenorphine. Arch Gen Psychiatry 35:501–516, 1978

Karan LD: Towards a broader view of recovery. J Subst Abuse Treat 10:101–105, 1993

Kaufman ER: Countertransference and other mutually interactive aspects of psychotherapy with substance abusers. American Journal on Addictions 1:185–202, 1992

Kaufman ER, Reoux J: Guidelines for the successful psychotherapy of substance abusers. Am J Drug Alcohol Abuse 14:199–209, 1988

Khantzian EJ: A contemporary psychodynamic approach to drug and alcohol treatment. Am J Drug Alcohol Abuse 12:213–222, 1986

Khantzian EJ, Halliday K, Golden S, et al: Modified group therapy for substance abusers. American Journal on Addictions 1:67–76, 1992

Leckman AL, Umland BE, Blay M: Prevalence of alcoholism in a family practice center. J Fam Pract 18:867–870, 1984

Leukefeld CG, Tims FM (eds): Drug Abuse Treatment in Prisons and Jails. National Institute on Drug Abuse Res Monograph 118 (DHHS Publ No ADM-92-1884). Washington, DC, US Government Printing Office, 1992

Magura S, Rosenblum A, Lewis C, et al: The effectiveness of in-jail methadone maintenance. Journal of Drug Issues 23:75–99, 1993

Manderscheid RW, Rae DS, Narrow WE, et al: Congruence of service utilization estimates from the epidemiologic catchment area project and other sources. Arch Gen Psychiatry 50:108–114, 1993

McLellan AT, Luborsky L, O'Brien CP, et al: Treatment in three different populations. Am J Drug Alcohol Abuse 12:101–120, 1987

McLellan AT, Arndt IO, Metzger DS, et al: The effects of psychosocial services in substance abuse treatment. JAMA 269:1953–1959, 1993

Mezzich J, Fabrega H, Coffman GA, et al: DSM-III disorders in a large sample of psychiatric patients. Am J Psychiatry 146:212–219, 1989

Moore RD, Bone LR, Geller G, et al: Prevalence, detection, and treatment of alcoholism in hospitalized patients. JAMA 261:403–407, 1989

Morton G: Central Texas Treatment Center, personal communication, June, 1993

National Consortium of Treatment Alternatives to Street Crime (TASC) Programs (eds): Providing Alcohol and Other Drug Treatment to Individuals in the Criminal Justice System Under National Health Care Reform. Washington, DC, National Consortium of Treatment Alternatives to Street Crime (TASC) Programs, June 1993

National Institute on Drug Abuse and National Institute on Alcohol Abuse and Alcoholism: 1989 Main Findings Report, National Drug and Alcoholism Treatment Unit Survey (NDATUS) (DHHS Publ No ADM-91-1729). Washington, DC, US Government Printing Office, 1990

Narrow WE, Regier DA, Rae DS, et al: Use of services by persons with mental and addictive disorders: findings from the National Institute of Mental Health Epidemiologic Catchment Area program. Arch Gen Psychiatry 50:95–107, 1993

O'Brien WB, Biase DV: Therapeutic community: a coming of age, in Substance Abuse: A Comprehensive Textbook, 2nd Edition. Edited by Lowinson JH, Ruiz P, Millman RB, et al. Baltimore, MD, Williams & Wilkins, 1992

Office of National Drug Control Policy: 1992 National Drug Control Strategy: A National Response to Drug Use. Washington, DC, US Government Printing Office, 1992

Orleans CT, George LK, Houpt JL, et al: How primary care physicians treat psychiatric disorders. Am J Psychiatry 142:52–57, 1985

Otto MW, Pollack MH, Sachs GS, et al: Discontinuance of benzodiazepine treatment. Am J Psychiatry 150:1485–1490, 1993

Persson J, Magnusson P: Prevalence of excessive or problem drinkers among patients attending somatic outpatient clinics: a study of alcohol related medical care. BMJ 295:467–472, 1987

Preventive Services Task Force: Guide to Clinic Preventive Services: An Assessment of the Effectiveness of 169 Interventions. Baltimore, MD, Williams & Wilkins, 1989

Pulver AE, Wolyniec PS, Wagner MG, et al: An epidemiologic investigation of alcohol dependent schizophrenics. Acta Psychiatr Scand 77:603–612, 1989

Regier D, Farmer ME, Rae DS, et al: Comorbidity of mental disorders with alcohol and other drug abuses. JAMA 264:2511–2518, 1990

Ridgeley MS, Goldman HH, Talbott JA: Chronic mentally ill young adults with substance abuse problems 1986, in Adolescent Psychiatry: Development and Clinical Studies. Edited by Feinstein SC. Chicago, IL, University of Chicago Press, 1989, pp 288–313

Scheier F, Siris S: A review of psychoactive substance use and abuse in schizophrenics. J Nerv Ment Dis 175:641–652, 1987

Schlesinger M, Dorwart RA: Falling between the cracks: failing national strategies for the treatment of drug abuse. Daedalus 121:195–238, 1992

Selzer ML: The Michigan Alcoholism Screening Test: the quest for a new diagnostic instrument. Am J Psychiatry 127:89–94, 1971.

Sternberg DE: Dual diagnosis: addiction and affective disorders. The Psychiatric Hospital 20(2):71–77, 1989

Substance Abuse and Mental Health Services Administration: Highlights From the 1991 National Drug and Alcoholism Treatment Unit Survey (NDATUS). Washington, DC, Substance Abuse and Mental Health Services Administration, September 1992a

Substance Abuse and Mental Health Services Administration, Office of Applied Studies: Preliminary Data From the 1992 NDATUS Study. Washington, DC, Substance Abuse and Mental Health Services Administration, 1992b

Swanson J, Morrissey JP, Goldstrom I, et al: Demographic and diagnostic characteristics of inmates receiving mental health services in state adult correctional
facilities: United States, 1988 (DHHS Publ No SMA-93-1995; Statistical Note
No 209). Washington, DC, U.S Government Printing Office, 1993

Swotinsky RB (ed): The Medical Review Officer's Guide to Drug Testing. New
York, Van Nostrand Reinhold, 1992

Tims FM (ed): Drug Abuse in Prisons. National Institute on Drug Abuse Treatment
Research Report Series (DHHS Publ No ADM-81-1149). Washington, DC, US
Government Printing Office, 1981

Vannicelli M: Removing the Roadblocks—Group Psychotherapy With Substance
Abusers and Family Members. New York, Guilford, 1992

Volpicelli JR, Alterman AI, Hayashida M, et al: Naltrexone in the treatment of
alcohol dependence. Arch Gen Psychiatry 49:876–880, 1992

Weiss RD, Mirin SM: The dual diagnosis alcoholic: evaluation and treatment.
Psychiatric Annals 19:261–265, 1989

Weiss RD, Stephens PS: Substance abuse and suicide, in Suicide and Clinical
Practice. Edited by Jacobs D. Washington, DC, American Psychiatric Press,
1992, pp 101–114

Whitemarsh GA, Thorward SR, Muller J: Profile of 1300 admissions to CNPHA-
CCRG hospitals. The Psychiatric Hospital 17:191–194, 1986

Wilens TE, O'Keefe JO, O'Connell JJ, et al: A public dual diagnosis detoxification
unit. American Journal on Addictions 2:91–98, 1993

Winokur G, Black D: Psychiatric and medical diagnoses as risk factors for
mortality in psychiatric patients. Am J Psychiatry 144:208–211, 1987

Woody GE, McLellan AT, Luborsky L, et al: Twelve months follow-up of
psychotherapy for opiate dependence. Am J Psychiatry 144:590–596, 1987

Zimberg S, Wallace J, Blume SB (eds): Practical Approaches to Alcoholism
Psychotherapy, 2nd Edition. New York, Plenum, 1985

Zweben JE, Payte JT: Methadone maintenance in the treatment of opioid dependence: a current perspective. West J Med 152:588–599, 1990

Chapter 3

Support for Addiction Treatment

Economic Issues

Cost of Addictive Diseases to American Society

Alcohol and other drug dependencies lead to devastating physical and psychological consequences for affected individuals, as discussed in Chapter 1. These personal costs are compounded by destructive effects on the families of those who are addicted: parents, spouses, offspring, and siblings. However, there is an additional dimension to the damage caused by addictive disorders, usually described as *societal cost*. Some aspects of societal cost cannot be measured in financial terms. These include the nation's morale, self-respect, and self-concept as a democratic and productive society. They also include fears of alcohol and other drug-related trauma on the highways and in the home, and fears of crime and violence related to the illicit drug trade. These concerns affect people's motivations and life decisions in ways that defy quantification.

Nevertheless, there are other aspects of the societal burden imposed by addictive diseases that can be expressed in dollars. In purely economic terms, the cost of addictive diseases to society greatly surpasses the cost to the affected individual (Cartwright and Kaple 1991a). A series of estimates of the societal cost were prepared for the National Institute on Alcohol Abuse and Alcoholism (NIAAA) and the National Institute on Drug Abuse (NIDA) (Harwood et al. 1984; Rice et al. 1990). Components of these cost estimates included medical costs, costs related to lost productivity, losses related to crime and costs to the criminal justice system, and costs related to special problems such as fetal alcohol syndrome and acquired immunodeficiency syndrome (AIDS). Overall estimates of substance-related costs during the years 1985–1988 were $70.3 billion in alcohol-related costs for 1985, which rose to $85.8 billion in constant dollars for 1988, and $44.1 billion in other drug-related costs (omitting tobacco) for 1985, which rose to $58.3 billion in constant dollars for 1988 (Rice et al. 1990).

In two recent reports, Parsons and Kamenca (1992, 1993) updated these estimates with 1991 figures and, assuming the persistence of current trends, projected costs to 1997. These estimates are summarized in Table 3–1 in comparison with the 1985 and 1988 costs, including the percentage of increases over the 1985 estimates. The rise in costs related to drug abuse-dependence was projected to be steeper than the rise of costs related to alcohol abuse-dependence, based on differences in the components of societal cost for these two categories, particularly the expenses that will accrue from the projected increase in drug-related cases of AIDS. About 29% of current AIDS cases are thought to have been contracted through intravenous drug use. The number of these individuals is projected to grow

Table 3–1. Estimated costs of alcohol- and other drug-related (excluding tobacco) problems to American society

	Alcohol-related problems	Other drug-related problems	Total
1985 estimate	$70.3 billion	$44.1 billion	$114.4 billion
1988 estimate Percentage increase above 1985 estimate	$85.8 billion 22.0%	$58.3 billion 32.1%	$144.1 billion 23.0%
1991 estimate Percentage increase above 1985 estimate	$91.9 billion 30.7%	$76.0 billion 72.3%	$167.9 billion 46.8%
1997 estimate Percentage increase above 1985 estimate	$123.8 billion 76.1%	$149.9 billion 239.9%	$273.7 billion 139.2%

Sources. Parsons and Kamenca 1993; Rice et al 1990.

by a factor of almost 6 between 1991 and 1997, with a proportional growth in the cost of their lost productivity and medical care. Thus, according to these projections, alcohol- and other drug-related problems will create $273.7 billion in social cost by 1997.

The estimates cited above have been criticized as imprecise, and various components of the overall cost have been criticized as being over- or underestimated, depending on the component being discussed (Department of Justice 1992; Heien and Pittman 1993; National Institute on Alcohol Abuse and Alcoholism 1991). However, although the precision of the figures may be imperfect, it remains true that, by any measurement, addiction-related problems are costly to society. It is also true that the effectiveness of attempts to decrease the prevalence of alcohol and other drug problems, through both prevention and treatment, can potentially be measured in economic as well as human terms.

In addition to the above cost estimates, various researchers have estimated the economic costs of tobacco use (including tobacco dependence) to the United States. In a 1993 report, the American Medical Association (AMA) estimated the current annual societal cost of tobacco use to be $85 billion, citing a 1985 report by the Office of Technology Assessment.

Looking specifically at the cost impact of addictive disorders within the health care system, it is evident that much of this cost is accounted for by treatment of the medical complications of the addictive disorder (e.g., trauma, hepatic cirrhosis), rather than treatment for the addiction itself. For example, in a general hospital survey of the cost of hospital stays for over 2,000 medical and surgical cases, Zook and Moore (1980) found that the highest cost 13% of patients consumed as many economic resources as the remaining 87%. Heavy drinking and smoking were more frequent among these patients. On any one day, approximately 25%–40% of patients in general hospital beds are there because of the complications of alcohol abuse-dependence (Holden 1987).

National concern has focused on the rising sum of health care expenditure and its increasing proportion to the country's total gross national product (GNP). According to the 1993 AMA report, in 1990 about $666.2 billion was spent on health care. During the 1980s, health care expenditures grew at an annual rate of 10.3%. As a percentage of the GNP, health care expenditures rose from 5.3% in 1960 to 9.2% in 1980 and 12.2% in 1990. The sources of financing for the health care system overall in 1990 were 57.5% private (32.5%, private insurance; 25%, out of pocket and other) and 42.4% government (29.3%, federal; 13.1%, state and local). Even though the contribution of private insurance has grown slowly and steadily in proportion to overall health care financing over the past 30 years (American Medical Association 1993), according to a report by Davis et al. (1990), the number of uninsured Americans has remained at about 37 million. This lack of access, combined with escalating costs, has created in the 1990s a climate of national will to achieve health system reform, both on state and national levels.

The 1993 AMA analysis of the growth in overall health care costs during the 1980s revealed that about 10% was a result of population growth, 69% was attributable to inflation (47% attributable to general inflation and 22%, to excess inflation of health care costs compared with others in the economy), and 21% was unexplained but said to be due to increasing volume (more services per capita) and intensity (use of more expensive services) (American Medical Association 1993). Addictive disorders are an important contributor to the high cost of health care. According to the 1993 AMA report, of the approximately 2 million deaths in the United States each year, about half are considered premature. Of these, nearly 60% are accounted for by tobacco use-dependence (434,000 deaths from direct use and 50,000 from environmental exposure to tobacco smoke or "passive smoking") and alcohol abuse-dependence (100,000 deaths annually). Rice et al. (1990) associated abuse-dependence of other drugs with an additional 6,100 deaths per year (Rice et al. 1990), not including drug-related deaths attributable to AIDS. Each tobacco-related death results in an average of 20 years lost from the normal expected life span; each alcohol-related death, 26 years; and each drug-related death, 37 years (Horgan et al. 1993). Clearly, if prevention and treatment are successful in reducing this excess mortality and its accompanying morbidity, an immediate relief of health care cost should result.

Financing of the Addiction Treatment System

History of financing. In this section, we focus on the network of organized services specializing in the treatment of substance use disorders (exclusive of nicotine). The sources of financing of this growing service system have shifted greatly during the last 40 years. Until the early 1970s, there were few such programs. For example, in a 1967 study, Plaut identified about 300 specialized alcoholism treatment programs in the United States. Each program was funded by resources specific to the facility (e.g., the Public Health Service drug treatment facilities and Veterans Administration programs were funded by the federal government; alcohol or drug programs based in state psychiatric hospitals were supported by state governments; municipal or county centers for detoxifying those found inebriated in public were funded by local governments). Private resources and charitable contributions supported private alcohol detoxification hospitals and residential rehabilitation units, as well as facilities for disadvantaged individuals, such as Salvation Army therapeutic residences for alcoholic individuals. Because health insurance coverage was generally unavailable to them, most indigent alcoholic patients received their medical care in emergency rooms and public hospitals. Those with insurance received care in community general hospitals, where they were admitted for the medical complications of alcoholism because these complications were covered by health insurance policies. Unfortunately, few were treated for their alcohol dependence. Those found drunk in public were often detoxified in jails. Indigent alcoholic individuals with chronic late-stage disease found their way in large numbers into state psychiatric facilities that lacked specialized alcoholism programs, where they received little more than custodial care. In the 1960s, as many as 40% of state psychiatric hospital admissions were patients with chronic alcoholism, although fewer than 10% of these hospitals had specialized alcoholism programs. Although private psychiatric hospitals also lacked specialized addiction treatment programs during the 1960s, alcoholism was identified as the major problem in only about 6% of their admissions (Institute of Medicine 1990).

Beginning in the late 1960s with respect to drug-specific facilities and in the early 1970s with respect to alcohol-specific facilities, the federal government assumed an increasing role in financing the development of the emerging publicly supported treatment system. This new funding developed along with a movement to separate public funding devoted to addictive disorder treatment programs from that devoted to mental health programs (Institute of Medicine 1990). With the help of federal grants and contracts in the 1970s, the states participated in a new federal-state partnership to develop networks of specialized addiction treatment in every community, according to need. Although state and local resources were used, by the late 1970s federal funds were the major public source of support for these programs. Each state identified a responsible state agency to plan the network and oversee the distribution of public funds. In 1976, public funds supported about 60% of the total cost of alcohol-related treatment and 91% of the total cost of other drug-related treatment (Gerstein and Harwood 1990). However, the federal-state balance began to shift in the 1980s with a decrease in federal participation and an increase in state responsibility for publicly funded treatment.

Also during the late 1970s and early 1980s, there was an increase in coverage of addiction treatment by both public and private health insurance plans. This effort to extend insurance coverage for such treatment to employees and their families, as well as to the publicly insured, was spearheaded by a series of federal and state initiatives. These initiatives included the development of an NIAAA model alcoholism benefit package in 1973 and NIAAA assistance to the states to promote employee assistance programs during the 1970s. Federal initiatives were coordinated with development efforts by state agencies, voluntary organizations (e.g., the National Council on Alcoholism and Drug Dependence labor-management initiatives), and the private sector (e.g., the Kemper Insurance Company [J. Miller et al. 1993]).

State legislatures around the country also considered measures to mandate minimum benefits for alcoholism and other drug treatment (Institute of Medicine 1990). Some of these measures required only that benefits be offered on a voluntary basis to all subscribers (i.e., *make available mandates*), whereas others required that a minimum benefit be provided. Nineteen states had some kind of insurance mandate in 1977, and 33 had one by 1982. In its 1990 study, the Institute of Medicine identified 37 states, plus the District of Columbia, that had health insurance mandates of some type: 19 for both alcoholism and other drug treatment coverage and 19 for alcoholism treatment alone. In 1981, the National Association of Insurance Commissioners added its weight to the movement when it adopted model legislation for the coverage of addictive disorders by group health insurance contracts and policies. Early studies on the effectiveness and cost-effectiveness of addiction treatment encouraged these developments.

Along with increases in addictive disease-specific coverage came a rapid increase in the number of specialized addiction treatment units in general and psychiatric hospitals. In 1986, the American Hospital Association identified 1,097 hospitals that reported having such units (Institute of Medicine 1990). Although many of the new facilities were in private, nonprofit settings, the for-profit sector also was growing rapidly. According to the 1991 National Drug and Alcoholism Treatment Unit Survey (NDATUS; Substance Abuse and Mental Health Services Administration 1992), among 9,034 addictive disorder treatment units reporting, 63.6% identified themselves as private, nonprofit organizations and 18.5% as private for-profit institutions, with the remaining 17.8% being owned by state-local (14.8%), federal (2.3%), or tribal (0.7%) governments.

The overall goal of these efforts to improve health insurance coverage was to move addiction treatment into the mainstream of health care financing. However, this goal was not fully attained for several reasons. First, the insurance coverage provided under state mandates included limits—on hospital or residential days, outpatient visits, numbers of treatment episodes, and total dollars expended—that were not applied to other types of mainstream medical care (except for psychiatric care) (Sharfstein et al. 1993). Second, many insurance plans were and still are exempt from state mandates. Public insurance programs (i.e., Medicare, Medicaid, and the Civilian Health and Medical Program of the Uniformed Services [CHAMPUS]) are exempt, as are many health maintenance organizations (HMOs). In addition, the Employment Retirement Income Security Act exempts self-insuring private corporations from mandates. As a result, self-insured companies have been found to be less likely to provide drug treatment coverage (other than for alcohol-related disorders) compared with plans subject to mandates, such as that of Blue Cross/Blue Shield (Gerstein and Harwood 1990). The evidence for a lower prevalence of alcoholism coverage among self-insured corporations is less clear (Institute of Medicine 1990).

To help identify differences between the financing of specialty alcoholism treatment and general health care, in its 1990 report the Institute of Medicine compared the available (though incomplete) data on financing for 1988 and 1989. Whereas direct state and local government funding accounted for 33% of alcoholism treatment financing, they accounted for only 8% of general health care financing. On the other hand, public health insurance accounted for 27% of general health care financing and only 8% of alcoholism treatment financing. The proportions of care financed by other sources was similar: direct federal funds—5% of alcoholism treatment, 7% of general health care; private health insurance—35% of alcoholism treatment, 32% of general health care; individual self-pay—14% of alcoholism treatment, 25% of general health care; and private donations or other funding—5% of alcoholism treatment, 2% of general health care.

With the growing national movement in the 1990s to legislate some type of health system reform at both the state and national levels, the configuration and adequacy of health insurance coverage for addictive disorders is again the subject of national debate. The version of reform finally adopted will have an overwhelming influence on the financing of all health services, but will have a particularly important effect on addiction treatment. The changes in financing will both dictate the accessibility of various addiction treatment modalities to people in need of help and potentially reshape the entire service system.

Current system financing.   There is no source available that provides a complete description of the current financing of the specialty addiction treatment network. A partial picture may be obtained from the White House's National Drug Control Strategy (Office of National Drug Control Policy 1992), from NDATUS (Substance Abuse and Mental Health Services Administration 1992), and from an additional study, the State Alcohol and Drug Abuse Profile (SADAP; Butinsky et al. 1991).

To place federal funds for the prevention and treatment of drug abuse-dependence (other than alcohol or nicotine) in the perspective of the federal government's war on drugs, we have shown in Figure 3–1 the proportions of federal funds devoted to domestic law enforcement and international and border control (i.e., *supply reduction*) versus those devoted to prevention and treatment of and research into drug addiction (i.e., *demand reduction*) (Office of National Drug Control Policy 1992). Although the overall amount of federal spending authorized to combat America's illegal drug epidemic has risen more than eightfold in 18 years, the proportion spent on demand reduction has changed relatively little. Since 1981, supply reduction programs have accounted for as much as 80% of the total budget, and never less than 70% (Reuter 1992).

The Office of National Drug Control Policy reported the combined budget authorizations requested for 1993 to support treatment and research as $2.3 billion, which represented 18.1% of the $12.7 billion total request.

In Table 3–2 we indicate how the 1991 federal funds actually authorized for treatment were distributed among federal agencies. The Alcohol, Drug Abuse, and Mental Health Administration showed the largest single expenditure of funds for treatment. In addition to the $800.6 million categorized for treatment, an additional $185.7 million, not reflected in Table 3–2, was classified as earmarked for treatment research. Of the $800.6 million allocated to treatment, $698.9 million was part of the federal block grant program, $83.3 million was for treatment improvement grants, $38.5 million was for waiting-list reduction grants, and the remainder was for other program grants. Of the estimated $190.5 million spent by the Health Care Financing Administration on drug treatment (exclusive of alcohol treatment), $130.5 million were Medicaid funds and $60.0 million were Medicare funds (including hospital costs only).

In the 1991 NDATUS survey, 7,480 alcoholism and other drug treatment units reported their source of financial support. A total of $4.14 billion was expended during the year on treatment; the percentages provided by different sources of funding are broken out in Table 3–3.

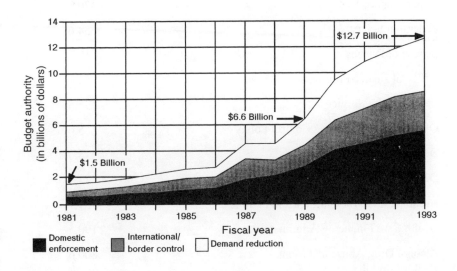

Figure 3–1. National drug control budget, 1981–1993.
Source. Office of National Drug Control Policy: *National Drug Control Strategy: A Nation Responds to Drug Use: Budget Summary.* Washington, DC, Executive Office of the President, 1992, p. 3.

In the SADAP study (Butinsky et al. 1991), only state programs that had received at least some funds administered by their alcohol-drug agency during the 1991 fiscal year were reported. Both prevention and treatment programs were included. In the report, 7,579 addiction treatment units were identified. This represented a number of units roughly comparable with that given in the NDATUS as state-local and nonprofit, but that is not to say both reports were referring to the identical units. In the SADAP study, $3.2 billion in funding was identified for prevention and treatment functions; the percentages provided by different sources of funding are broken out in Table 3–4. Approximately $2.4 billion, or 75% of the total, was allocated to treatment units (Butinsky et al. 1991).

Like the NDATUS, the SADAP presented only a partial picture of the state-local treatment network financing. When asked to estimate what

Table 3–2.   Federal support for drug treatment in 1991

Department	Funds received (in millions of dollars)
Department of Veterans Affairs	470.9
Federal judiciary	34.6
Bureau of Prisons	10.7
Office of Justice Programs	83.1
Indian Health Service	35.3
Office of National Drug Control Policy	5.6
Department of Defense	15.0
Department of Education	74.1
Administration for Children and Families	31.7
Health Care Financing Administration	190.5
Alcohol Drug Abuse and Mental Health Administration (for programs now administered by SAMHSA)	800.6
Total	1,752.1

Source.   Office of National Drug Control Policy 1992.

Table 3–3. Source of funds for alcoholism and other drug treatment units, 1991

Source of funds	Percentage of total financing of treatment system
Federal block grant funds	7.9
Federal grant funds (exclusive of block grant program)	6.4
State and local grants (exclusive of block grant program)	34.2
Public and private third-party payment	33.4
Private insurance	21.2
Medicaid	8.9
Medicare	2.2
Other public third parties	1.1
Client fees	10.8
Public welfare funds	2.3
Private donations	1.7
Other or unknown sources	3.3

Source. Substance Abuse and Mental Health Services Administration 1992.

Table 3–4. State and local funds expended on alcoholism and drug treatment, 1991

Source of funds	Percentage of total funds expended in state-local treatment system
Federal block grant funds	29.2
Other federal agencies	8.5
Direct state funds (through state alcohol/drug agency)	34.4
Other state agencies	5.2
County or other local agencies	6.9
Other sources (including Medicaid, insurance, client fees)	15.5

Source. Butinsky et al. 1991.

percentage of the state's total addiction treatment system was represented by the programs reported in the SADAP (i.e., the state-administered funds-assisted programs), the states and territories provided estimates varying from 100% in Guam and Puerto Rico to 30% in North Dakota and 31.8% in Colorado. Although Minnesota estimated that 95% of its programs were included, Texas estimated only 41%. Thus, an important, but unknown, segment of the treatment network is not reflected in these data. Among these programs are units supported entirely by private insurance and private donations and facilities funded entirely by federal or tribal funds such as Department of Veterans Affairs–sponsored units, Indian Health programs, and United States military treatment programs.

In an effort to estimate the cost of a comprehensive addiction treatment benefit under national health care reform, Harwood et al. (1994) applied a series of corrections and adjustments to data derived from the 1991 NDATUS report to produce a service utilization and cost estimate for 1993. Corrections were made for study nonresponse by treatment units, inflation, and underinclusion of community mental health centers. In addition, estimates of $47 million for the cost of visits to physicians, $29 million for visits to psychologists, and $13 million for visits to social workers in private practice were added to the total. Having made these adjustments, Harwood et al. estimated that, in 1993, approximately 3 million individuals participated in a total of 5.8 million treatment episodes, at a total cost of $6.7 billion. In terms of the number of treatment episodes, about 10% took place in hospitals; 7%, in freestanding detoxification facilities; 16%, in residential care; and 67%, in outpatient settings. In terms of total expenditure, inpatient hospital care accounted for 25.5% of the total expenditure; freestanding detoxification, 3.7%; residential care, 30%; and outpatient treatment, about 40.8%.

Harwood et al. (1994) further estimated that, for 1993, $4.33 billion of public funds, $1.63 billion of private insurance funds, and $770 million of user payments supported treatment for alcohol and other drug disorders. The national average of spending per covered life was $25.75, with $45.70 per life for individuals covered by the public sector and $13.55 by the private sector. The cost of a comprehensive addiction treatment benefit for all Americans in need of such services was estimated at $45.10 per covered life per year. This would provide approximately 6.3 million treatment episodes to 3.3 million individuals annually.

Effectiveness and Cost-Benefit
Profile of Addiction Treatment

Having examined the prevalence and societal cost of the psychoactive substance use disorders and the nature, extent, and financing of the current addiction treatment network, we now turn to a consideration of current knowledge about the effectiveness of these treatments. Related research questions concern their cost-benefit profile, cost-effectiveness, and cost offsets. A *cost-benefit analysis* is a comparison of the financial cost of a treatment episode and its resultant benefits, expressed in money saved, lives saved, or other terms. *Cost-effectiveness* gives the ratio of the relative costs and benefits (expressed in financial terms) of different types or settings of treatment for equivalent patient populations. *Cost offset* is a comparison of the costs of treatment with the savings produced within the health care system itself by the reduced need for medical services among individuals who received that treatment.

Studies of the effectiveness of treatment for substance use disorders have been conducted over the past 50 years. Treatment outcome studies are the most common type of research, with an estimated 600 published studies of alcoholism treatment alone, about half published since 1980. In addition, about 200 comparative clinical trials of alcoholism treatment, many using a random assignment design, have been completed (Institute of Medicine 1990). Likewise, documented in the scientific literature are the results of many outcome studies of treatment for other drug dependence, including methadone treatment, drug-free outpatient treatment, therapeutic communities, and prison-based programs (Cartwright and Kaple 1991b; Gerstein and Harwood 1990; Pickens et al. 1991). Authors reviewing these studies have generally concluded that treatments are effective—that is, they yield a better outcome than the absence of treatment (Cartwright and Kaple 1991b; Emrick 1975; Gerstein and Harwood 1990; Gottheil et al. 1992; Hubbard et al. 1989; Institute of Medicine 1989, 1990; Jones and Vischi 1979; McLellan et al. 1991; National Association of Addiction Treatment Providers 1991; National Association of State Alcohol and Drug Abuse Directors 1990; Pickens et al. 1991; Saxe et al. 1983). However, it has also been pointed out in these reviews that general questions of effectiveness must be refined. The more pertinent question to ask is, Which treatments are most effective for which subgroups of addicted patients?

This question can only be answered through studies of clearly specified clinical populations that use precisely described treatment methods, define standard outcome measures (verified by chemical tests and collateral sources whenever possible), and are conducted by disinterested researchers. Although randomized controlled trials are perhaps the most useful way to measure relative efficacy, they are costly and difficult to conduct. Outcome studies monitoring pre- and posttreatment variables, particularly those tracking large patient populations, also contribute a great deal to current knowledge.

Another important contribution of long-term follow-up studies has been the understanding that, for most addicted people, treatment is not a single event. Significant improvement following a treatment episode may be followed by later relapse, which again responds to treatment. Recovery techniques learned over the course of several treatments may finally result in long-term stable remission. It is therefore somewhat misleading to credit the recovery of an individual patient to his or her last treatment episode and thereby consider all previous treatment episodes to have failed. Addictive disorders must be understood as chronic and relapsing diseases, although long-term recovery is attainable. In structuring both a network of treatment services and a health insurance benefit for addictive disorders, the use of an acute illness-acute care model is inappropriate.

One important large scale longitudinal study of addiction was the Treatment Outcome Prospective Study (Hubbard et al. 1989), a multiyear follow-up of nearly 10,000 individuals treated in 37 programs in different parts of the United States. The 12 outpatient methadone, 14 residential therapeutic community, and 11 drug-free outpatient facilities included in the study specialized in treating addicted patients whose primary dependence was to a drug other than alcohol or nicotine. Patients admitted during the years 1979–1981 were followed for up to 5 years. Substantial and significant improvement in status was found for patients treated in all modalities studied. In addition, reductions in alcohol and other drug use, reductions in criminal activity, and improvements in functional capacity were found.

Another example of a large multisite outcome study system is the Comprehensive Assessment and Treatment Outcome Research (CATOR) program, a privately funded independent evaluation service. As of 1992, 38 inpatient and 19 outpatient chemical dependency–model, abstinence-based programs were being monitored (Hoffman and Miller 1992). Data on the nearly 10,000 generally middle-class, seriously affected patients treated in these programs were used to calculate 6-month and 1-year abstinence rates following treatment, using best- and worst-case assumptions about patients lost to follow-up. For former inpatients, between 50% and 66.7% attained stable abstinence at 6 months and between 34% and 60% at 12 months. For outpatients, between 57% and 75% attained stable abstinence at 6 months and between 42% and 68% at 1 year. Abstinence was accompanied by improvement in health, social, and economic functioning.

Research studies spanning many years have elucidated factors that predict successful treatment outcome. These factors include patient-specific variables such as severity of illness, comorbid medical and psychiatric conditions, age, gender, and degree of social stability (e.g., marital status, employment status, residence). Important treatment variables include the type, duration, and intensity of treatment provided (Cartwright and Kaple 1991b; Filstead 1989a, 1989b; Gibbs and Flanagan 1977; Gottheil et al. 1992; McLellan et al. 1991, 1993; National Association of Addiction Treatment Providers 1991). In addition, posttreatment life events, life stresses, coping strategies, and social supports were found to play a significant role in outcome (Finney and Moos 1992).

Naturalistic evaluation and random assignment studies have recently been complemented by studies that concentrate on patient-treatment matching (Finney and Moos 1986; Gerstein and Harwood 1990; Glaser 1980; Institute of Medicine 1989, 1990). These studies promise to refine current knowledge about differential treatment effectiveness.

Costs versus benefits.   Investigators attempting to understand the costs of addiction treatment in comparison to its benefits have used many approaches, most of which have shown positive results. One way to measure costs versus benefits is in the number of lives saved. The high mortality rates associated with alcoholism have been alluded to above. Several long-term outcome studies have shown that treated alcoholic patients (Barr et al. 1984; Bullick et al. 1992; Smith et al. 1983) and other drug-addicted individuals (Barr et al. 1984) who have achieved abstinence attain mortality rates expected for their age and gender, whereas those who failed to recover experienced excess mortality. Although this saving of life has not been expressed in relationship to treatment costs (i.e., cost per additional person-year of life), such a cost-benefit figure might be calculated.

A common approach to cost-benefit analysis has been measurement of decreased criminal behavior following treatment for addiction and translation of that reduction into decreased societal cost (Gerstein and Harwood 1990). Follow-up from the Treatment Outcome Prospective Study project has been used to calculate the dollar cost to society of study patients during the year before and the year after the index treatment episode, including criminal justice costs (Hubbard et al. 1989). Depending on the components of cost included in the estimates and the method of calculation, the benefit-to-cost ratio of these programs ranged from 0.92 to 4.28. Thus, the benefit to society ranged from nearly equal to the cost of treatment to more than 4 times greater.

Results of studies measuring costs versus benefits in dollars for alcoholism treatment have been particularly positive in employment-based populations referred by employee assistance programs. For example, in a cost-benefit analysis of the Navy's alcoholism rehabilitation program, Borthwick (1977) concluded that discharging and replacing diagnosed alcoholic service members would cost 2.2 times more than the cost of their treatment. The Navy spent $22.6 million on treatment of Navy and Marine Corps personnel, whereas replacing the number of person-years of service salvaged would have cost $49 million.

In a similar study evaluating the cost of the Navy's residential alcohol-drug facilities (both freestanding and based at naval hospitals) versus the cost of replacing personnel, Caliber Associates (1989) found that the Navy's overall treatment program yielded a benefit-to-cost ratio of 12.9:1, with alcohol treatment at 13.8:1, other drug treatment at 10.3:1, and poly-drug treatment at 6.8:1.

Treatment populations of employed individuals were studied by several corporations in the 1970s (Jones and Vischi 1979). One example was the study done for the Illinois Bell Corporation, in which 402 employees were followed for 5 years after alcoholism treatment. At that point, 57% were continuously abstinent for more than 1 year and another 15% had improved in comparison to their original status. Sickness and disability days were reduced by 46%; off-duty accidents, by 63%; and on-duty accidents, by 81%. In a study from General Motors of Canada, 104 treated alcoholic employees showed a 48% reduction in benefit use and 64% drop in workers' compensation compared with 48 untreated alcoholic employees, who showed a 127% increase in benefit use and 79% increase in workers' compensation.

Another example of cost-benefit analysis was Cartwright and Kaple's (1991) study of patients whose methadone treatment was interrupted by the closing of a clinic. They compared patients who continued treatment by transferring to another clinic with those who did not. Annual cost to the community was higher for those who did not continue treatment ($10,982 for male patients, $9,689 for female patients) than for those who transferred to further treatment ($4,031 for male patients and $3,881 for female patients). The higher costs mainly reflected crime-related and criminal justice system costs.

An additional factor in the societal cost related to addictive disorders is the spread of AIDS. Costs for treatment of patients with injection-drug–related AIDS are expected to accelerate over the next few years. Thus, one future approach to cost-benefit analysis of addiction treatment is to base evaluations of the effectiveness of treatment on the primary prevention of AIDS. Considerations important for such research were discussed in a recent NIDA monograph (Cartwright and Kaple 1991b).

Cost-effectiveness. Considerations of cost-effectiveness are of great interest in the debate over health care reform, particularly in relation to publicly financed programs. The state of Oregon adopted a radical approach to reform of its Medicaid system in a 5-year experiment approved by its legislature in 1993. Using a modified cost-effectiveness approach, the Oregon Health Services Commission ranked more than 700 medical treatments in order of priority, with the most cost-effective and socially valuable treatments at the top of the list (i.e., treatments of acute fatal conditions that lead to full recovery). Under the new program, Medicaid coverage is extended to thousands of uninsured people, but only treatments ranking above a cut-off level determined by funding considerations are covered. Although mental health and addiction services will be phased into the plan at a later date than will other medical services, the treatment of addictive disorders was ranked 154th, well above any proposed cut-off level (J. Miller et al. 1993). Reviews of many other public sector cost-effectiveness studies can be found in the literature (Cartwright and Kaple 1991b; Gerstein and Harwood 1990; Institute of Medicine 1989, 1990; Jones and Vischi 1979; Saxe et al. 1983).

Cost-effectiveness has also been explored in private sector studies. In their 1991 report, Walsh et al. compared costs and outcome for 227 employees referred for alcoholism treatment by the employee assistance program of a large New England company. These employees were randomly assigned to three treatment groups:

1. Compulsory inpatient treatment, with participation in Alcoholics Anonymous (AA) following discharge
2. Compulsory participation in AA alone
3. A free choice among inpatient treatment, outpatient treatment, participation in AA, or a combination of treatment and an AA program

Only "gray area" cases (i.e., patients not obviously in need of hospital or noninpatient care) were included in the study. The compulsory inpatient group had the best outcome over a 2-year period, measured in terms of alcohol and drug use. The group exercising free choice did next best, and the compulsory AA group did the least well. This difference was particularly true for employees who had a history of cocaine abuse-dependence. Because the AA-alone and free-choice groups required more inpatient admissions following the index referral, total treatment costs of these groups were approximately 90% of the cost of the group initially referred to inpatient care.

Cost offset.   Perhaps the most immediately useful research for understanding the direct value of addiction treatment within the mainstream of health care is cost offset research. These studies examine the cost of treatment specific to a substance use disorder in relationship to costs incurred by the same patients within the general health care system both before and after addiction treatment. Such studies have been reported primarily in relation to the treatment of alcohol abuse-dependence (Blose and Holder 1991; Holder 1987).

It is well established that individuals who abuse or are dependent on alcohol incur much higher medical costs than nonalcoholic control groups during the years before they enter alcoholism treatment (Blose and Holder 1991). It is interesting that costs of medical care for the families of alcoholic individuals are also significantly higher than average. In one study (Blose and Holder 1991), these costs were double the per-person costs in control families.

The utilization and cost of general health care services for the alcoholic patient, particularly in general hospital inpatient treatment, increases steeply during the year before alcoholism-specific treatment is initiated (Holder and Blose 1992). On the other hand, results from outcome studies following large numbers of patients after discharge from addiction treatment (e.g., Hoffman and Miller 1992) have demonstrated significant decreases in general hospital admissions and emergency room visits during the year after treatment compared with the year before. Similarly, results from employment-based studies have documented decreases in days away from work attributable to illness, injury, and hospitalization following treatment (Jones and Vischi 1979). These findings can be converted into cost offset estimates (Holder 1987).

Two large-scale studies of this kind have recently been reported by Holder and Blose (1986, 1992). In their 1986 study, these researchers analyzed the health care utilization costs of 1,697 federal employees treated for alcoholism (77% treated as inpatients with an average stay of 22 days). The cost of their claims rose steeply before treatment, fell during the first posttreatment year, and continued to drop during the following year. This drop was especially marked in those age 44 years or less at the time of treatment. In this group, average monthly health care costs fell progressively during the 36 months following treatment, falling to the level comparable with the total monthly costs incurred 36 months prior to the alcoholism treatment, despite the fact that these individuals were now 6 years older (Holder and Blose 1986).

In their 1992 study, Holder and Blose extended the original findings using two separate research designs. The authors analyzed a database of 20 million health care claims for 260,000 insurance plan enrollees (white- and blue-collar workers and families, some of whom belonged to HMOs). These claims covered a 14-year period and allowed a comparison between enrollees treated for alcoholism and enrollees treated for alcohol-related complications only. In the study, the authors identified 3,068 alcoholic individuals who received alcoholism treatment and 661 who were treated only for complications of the disease. They again found that health costs fell considerably after treatment for alcoholism, declining by 23%–55% below pretreatment levels. Untreated alcoholic individuals, on the other hand, incurred health care costs that were 24% higher than those for treated alcoholic individuals, even though the costs of the alcoholism treatment itself were included in the totals for the treated group (Holder and Blose 1992).

Pre- and posttreatment comparisons of health care costs, as well as comparisons of other negative consequences of addictive disorders, are often criticized as confounding treatment effects with statistical regression to the mean. The long period of time included in the Holder and Blose studies (Holder and Blose 1986, 1992) and the time series analysis used (Holder and Blose 1992) make this explanation unlikely.

The statistical regression hypothesis has been further tested in an analysis of health care costs for 3,572 adult inpatients treated for substance use disorders and tracked for 2 years in the CATOR program (Hoffman et al. 1993). About half of the patients were treated for alcohol problems only, whereas the rest reported both alcohol and other drug (other than nicotine) use. Recovery, defined as total abstinence during the entire 2-year follow-up period, was reported to have been attained by 58.8% of the patients. The other patients, who had experienced at least one relapse, were considered not in recovery. Although the two groups did not differ in the number of inpatient hospitalization days in the 12 months before addiction treatment, they differed significantly in number of inpatient hospitalization days during both the first and second posttreatment year. By the second year, inpatient hospital utilization for patients who had at least one relapse rose to within 80% of pretreatment levels (35% below pretreatment rates the first year and 19% below pretreatment rates the second year). For recovering patients, these rates remained well under half of the pretreatment levels (61% below pretreatment rates the first year and 57% below pretreatment rates the second year). Making the extreme assumption that addiction treatment had no effect at all on the group with at least one relapse, excess hospital care because of pretreatment crises would not account for more than 20% of the total, and regression to the mean could not account for more than a small portion of the decreased posttreatment inpatient hospitalization. In fact, many of these relapsed patients had greatly reduced their alcohol-drug use, and about 45% of them had a full year of abstinence during the 2-year follow-up period. Thus, much of their decreased hospitalization was also attributable to treatment. The authors of the study concluded that addiction treatment in this population produced large and sustained cost offsets within the health care system.

Despite vastly different populations and methodologies, the majority of studies of treatment for addictive disorders have shown treatment to be effective, cost beneficial, and productive of cost offsets within the health care system.

Addiction Treatment Financing Through Insurance

Insurance Coverage for Addictive Disorders

As discussed in the section "Financing of the Addiction Treatment System," above, the provision of health insurance coverage for addictive disorders has been a relatively recent phenomenon. Although such coverage is currently widespread, insurers still consider addiction treatment coverage to be an "add-on" or "fringe" benefit, rather than an integral part of any basic health insurance package (Institute of Medicine 1990).

At present, in the United States, more than 150 million people are covered by private health insurance—in most cases, insurance obtained through their employment or as a family member of an employed person (Gerstein and Harwood 1990). In private industry, an increasing number of plans offer coverage for substance use disorders. For example, according to Gerstein and Harwood (1990), 36% of medium- to large-size employers (i.e., those with more than 100 employees) provided alcoholism coverage in 1981, a rate that rose to 68% in 1985 and 86% in 1988. Furthermore, for drug addiction treatment, the proportions of medium- to large-size companies offering this coverage were 43% in 1983, 66% in 1985, and 74% in 1988. A larger proportion of HMO than non-HMO plans provided some form of drug treatment coverage.

Results from surveys of public employee benefits have indicated that some form of addiction treatment coverage is universally available to federal employees and only slightly less so to state and local employees (Gerstein and Harwood 1990). As of 1988, the federal government provided health insurance to approximately 4 million employees, covering nearly 10 million people (including employees and families). Every federal employee plan is required to include some coverage for substance use disorder treatment, but no specific minimum is required (Gerstein and

Harwood 1990). Results from a 1987 survey of state and local government employee plans indicated that approximately 94% of the 10.3 million full-time state and local government employees received health insurance benefits (Bureau of Labor Statistics 1987). Of these, 94% had some type of addiction treatment benefit.

In many employee benefit plans, the addiction treatment coverage is combined with that for mental health, but in others, addiction treatment benefits are specified separately and may be provided at different levels. However, similar to the restrictions on mental health coverage, addiction treatment generally is subject to discriminatory coverage, with co-payments or deductibles; limits on number of visits, length of stay, and number of inpatient days; and sometimes dollar payment caps not imposed on other medical care (Sharfstein et al. 1993). In addition, many plans limit their inpatient treatment benefits to detoxification only, making continued inpatient or residential intensive treatment unavailable. According to Gerstein and Harwood's (1990) report, this was true for 20% of employees of medium- and large-size companies with some addiction coverage in 1989. Also, many policies do not have provisions for intensive outpatient or partial hospitalization services, thereby encouraging the use of more expensive inpatient treatment for some patients who might otherwise profit from day or evening programs. This was true for 16% of employees of medium- and large-size companies with some addiction coverage in 1989 (Gerstein and Harwood 1990).

Typical limits on mental health and addiction coverage are illustrated by the findings of a 1989 survey of 976 private employers (average work force, 7,642 employees) (Hewitt Associates 1990). Nearly all plans ($n = 933$) reported special limits on mental health and addiction treatment coverage. The patterns of limitation varied widely, with in- and outpatient limits differing. The typical patterns found were an annual limit for alcohol or drug inpatient care of $2,500, a limit of 30 days of care, and a lifetime limit of $10,000. For outpatient care, the typical constraints included an annual limit of 50 visits, a maximum of $35 per visit, an annual limit of $1,000, and a lifetime limit of $10,000. In addition, cost-management measures were common, including precertification (54% of plans), concur-rent utilization review (49% of plans), case management (58% of plans), outpatient incentives (13% of plans), use of a preferred provider organization (10% of plans), and use of a psychiatric HMO (6% of plans).

Typical policies for local and state government employees also imposed special limitations on addiction treatment not imposed on other health care. This was true for 71% of state and local government employees who had some coverage for alcohol or drug treatment. Inpatient days were characteristically limited to 30/year, and dollar caps were imposed. Outpatient limits also were more stringent than constraints on other ambulatory medical care. This was true for 84% of employees with outpatient addiction coverage. Visits were limited to 30–50 visits/year, higher co-payments were required, and dollar caps were imposed (Gerstein and Harwood 1990).

Federal employees' plans were found to vary considerably, but tended to favor inpatient care. As of 1988, typical fee-for-service plans offered $4,000–$6,000/year for addiction treatment, with significant deductibles and co-payments. Of all plans surveyed, 22% had no outpatient benefit at all, and an additional 30% limited outpatient payments to $250–$400/year (Gerstein and Harwood 1990).

Benefit Utilization

Ford (1992) studied utilization rates for private insurance addiction benefits (including Blue Cross/Blue Shield) as reflected in the MEDSTAT database of 3.6 million insured individuals' claims for 1989 and 1990. Ninety-five percent of individuals in the study had coverage for 30 days or more of inpatient care, and more than half had no outpatient limit on visits. Addiction treatment inpatient admissions accounted for 3.4% of all hospital admissions in 1989 and 2.7% in 1990. Addiction inpatient care accounted for 3.8% of all payments for inpatient stays in 1989 and 3% in 1990. The cost per insured person was $22.37 for the year 1989 and $17.70 in 1990. The average cost of an inpatient stay for addiction treatment was about $470/day for an average of 18 days (total $8,500), compared with an average inpatient stay for psychiatric treatment of 21.4 days at $640/day (total $13,700). Outpatient addiction treatment accounted for 0.6% of all outpatient costs in 1989 and 0.4% in 1990. The annual cost was $3.14 per insured person in 1989 and $2.42 in 1990.

It is interesting that Ford (1992) documented a decrease in inpatient admissions between 1989 and 1990, despite adequate levels of inpatient benefits. This drop was attributed to cost-containment measures, particularly those used in managed care. Such a decrease in inpatient care would presumably indicate that potential inpatients were referred to outpatient care as a less costly option. However, the fact that there was also a drop in outpatient treatment costs raises doubts that this transfer actually occurred. The major finding of Ford's (1992) study was that addiction treatment itself, as contrasted with the treatment of the complications of substance use disorders, is not a major factor in the overall cost of privately insured health care coverage.

Other researchers have looked at combined psychiatric and addiction treatment utilization. In a report by the Hay/Huggins Company (1992), the structure of coverage for psychiatric and addiction care was compared with that of nonpsychiatric care coverage for 1,048 employers. Similar disparities to those mentioned above were documented. Psychiatric and addiction care were found to account for about 8% of these employers' total health care costs for 1991. The annual cost for psychiatric and addiction coverage in an average plan was $156/employee or $408/family, or about 8% of the total costs. Hay/Huggins further calculated the additional cost of bringing the levels of psychiatric and addiction treatment and other medical care benefits to parity in various benefit packages; the costs for doing so ranged from $36/year to $96/year for an individual employee and from $96/year to $264/year for a family.

One final consideration in understanding the utilization of private insurance coverage is its relation to publicly supported care. Health insurance coverage for psychiatric and addiction treatment, as it is widely applied today, provides what is meant to be a basic benefit adequate to cover the needs of most subscribers. This basic benefit structure does not include comprehensive coverage for extended, severe illnesses (so-called catastrophic coverage). For such care, individuals with only basic insurance coverage are obliged to pay out of pocket, and, if personal resources are insufficient, to rely on public sector or charity facilities (Sharfstein et al. 1993). Thus, limitations on insurance benefits and those cost-containment measures that curtail access to care may result in the shifting of costs from the private to the public sector—that is, the "dumping" of underinsured patients into the already crowded public system.

Systems of Cost Containment

Parity in benefits between general medical and addiction treatment would be of little consequence if individuals in need of care were unable to access treatment. Recent concerns about excessive limits on access to care have focused not only on the structure of the addiction treatment benefit, but also on the care management system accompanying the benefit. Despite the relatively small proportion of total health care fiscal resources devoted to psychiatric and addiction treatment, insurers and corporations view this segment of the health care system with some anxiety. There is a fear the system will be abused—not only by the few unscrupulous providers who intentionally provide unnecessary care, but by the treatment system as a whole. The treatment of substance use disorders, like the treatment of other mental disorders, is looked on as a "soft" area of medicine in which judgments are more difficult to quantify and more subjective than in other medical or surgical care. In addition, there is a fear of the potential for long-term or custodial care. The development of patient placement criteria (e.g., Hoffman et al. 1991) and practice guidelines (e.g., the *Practice Guideline for Substance Use Disorders* currently being developed by the American Psychiatric Association) has made some headway in helping those concerned with containing health costs understand the contemporary practice of addiction treatment. However, doubts remain.

The perceived need for special cost controls in the mental and substance use disorder segment of health care has been the major motivation for the array of limits and restrictions on insurance coverage and benefit utilization. Demand for addiction services has also been considered to be more "price elastic" than that for general medical care; a lower direct cost to the patient is thought to increase the demand for services and therefore the utilization of benefits. Better research on addiction treatment is needed to test this hypothesis (Gerstein and Harwood 1990). However, Hayami and Freeborn (1981), in their study of 250 patients treated for alcoholism within the Kaiser Permanente Medical Care Program, Oregon Region, did not find this prediction to be accurate. They compared 134 patients whose care was subject to a 50% co-payment with 116 patients who had full coverage. There was no difference in the decrease in total medical utilization, but the group without a co-payment made more alcoholism treatment contacts, and improved somewhat more in drinking behavior and abstinence. Statistical analysis found the difference in benefit limits a relatively unimportant factor in treatment outcome.

In addition to the various types of benefit limits, structural systems of cost containment have been instituted (Gerstein and Harwood 1990; Institute of Medicine 1990). These include the provision of services in organizational systems other than the traditional fee-for-service insurance reimbursement model (e.g., in HMOs). For the larger number of providers who are not part of such a system, cost containment has meant the institution of various forms of case management, including preadmission certification, concurrent utilization review, retrospective review, provider profiling, and program audits.

Case management.   The term *case management* is currently used in two senses. Case management was originally developed as a component in the care of chronically ill individuals who needed a variety of medical, rehabilitative, and social services. This *facilitator model* case manager functions independently of any specific treatment payer or provider, acting as a patient advocate and facilitating the patient's access to needed services (Willenbring et al. 1991). The case manager can also potentially bring cost savings to the health and human services systems by keeping the patient with multiple problems connected with needed services, preventing relapse or the need for rehospitalization, and choosing the most cost-effective level of care. However, the cost containment success of the facilitator model is determined by both the availability and accessibility of various components of the needed continuum of care, as well as the structure of available finances.

The second case management model, the *gatekeeper model,* is the case management process currently in use throughout much of the health care system. The goal of this style of management is to manage access to various services through controlling lengths of stay and favoring lower cost treatment wherever feasible. This model case manager does not function independently, but rather is an agent of the payer and thus has built-in incentives to reduce overall costs. This creates the potential for generating savings by refusing to pay for levels of care that are needed, based on inappropriate or arbitrary criteria; for example, a case manager may refuse to approve inpatient care unless a prospective patient has failed at an "adequate trial" of outpatient care within a given period of time, or the case manager may insist on a level of care for which the individual has no benefits or which is currently unavailable. Clinicians working with addicted patients have reacted with alarm to the recent proliferation of case management systems within the health care system (J. B. Cutler, American

Psychiatric Association Division of Government Relations, unpublished letter to Mrs. Tipper Gore, May 1993; Legal Action Center 1992). Complaints by addiction treatment clinicians include denial of access to needed care, the use of case managers untrained in addiction treatment, inconsistencies in definitions of medical necessity and refusal by managers to reveal their criteria for medical necessity (considering this proprietary information), inadequate appeals processes, unwarranted demands for sensitive patient information, and excessive and unnecessary burdens of telephone time and paperwork.

In theory, organized case management can 1) ensure that each patient in need of treatment is matched with the most appropriate and least restrictive level of care, 2) minimize patients' delay in reaching treatment, and 3) track the patients' progress and treatment outcome through decreasing levels of treatment intensity. The data thus acquired can, in turn, enable the system to profile the effectiveness and efficiency of each provider. These profiles can be useful in curtailing excess utilization and containing costs. Working at its best, managed care does accomplish some of these goals. Working less than optimally, the system causes problems to providers and patients alike.

Because of problems within newly developed case management systems, state legislatures have considered, and in some cases have passed, measures to regulate external utilization review organizations. The goals of these regulations are to ensure at least a minimum level of staff qualifications, the adequacy of decision-making criteria, the system's accessibility to patients, the adequacy of appeal procedures, and the protection of sensitive personal information (General Accounting Office 1992; Willenbring et al. 1991).

HMOs, preferred provider organizations (PPOs), and independent practice associations (IPAs) are increasingly popular models of care management. Other models are primary care case management, in which a primary care provider (usually a physician) must authorize all referrals to specialty care, and contracting by a health insurance organization with a fiscal intermediary to arrange for and pay for covered services (Macro International 1992).

Health maintenance organizations. In 1973, the federal HMO act was passed, which provided grants, loans, and loan guarantees to stimulate the development of HMOs. The goal of this legislation was to encourage the provision of prepaid health care on a capitated basis as an alternative to traditional fee-for-service care. HMOs typically use salaried clinicians (as in the staff model HMO) or networks of private practitioners and institutions with whom they have contracted. The contract between the providers and an HMO usually involves some form of financial risk sharing and the use of a case management system.

According to a 1993 report from the Health Insurance Association of America, in 1992 about one-quarter of the 47% of insured American workers subject to managed care were enrolled in HMOs, with an additional 22% enrolled in PPOs or similar plans. The HMO act of 1973 mandated the inclusion of some addiction treatment services in federally qualified HMOs. However, the mandate required "medical treatment and referral," with no specified minimum coverage. About 5% of HMO total medical care costs are spent on mental health and addiction treatment combined. In their 1982 survey of 205 HMOs, Levin and Glasser (1984) found that more than half offered care for alcoholism and other drug treatment, whereas in a similar survey conducted in 1986, two-thirds offered such care (Levin et al. 1988).

Results of a more recent study by Levin (1993) that included 17 HMOs, representing over 2.2 million enrollees nationwide, indicated that all HMOs had some addiction treatment coverage, but that the nature of the benefits varied considerably both between HMOs and within them, depending on subscriber contracts. Most plans excluded methadone maintenance and long-term inpatient rehabilitation treatment (i.e., more than 30 days). In many HMOs, mental health and addiction services were provided together. Within HMOs that provided addiction treatment services, the average staff ratio was one mental health or addiction professional per 5,000 enrollees. HMOs with separate addiction services reported that these services were staffed with psychiatrists, psychologists, nurses, or addiction counselors. About 18% of the addiction-specific staff were psychiatrists. Utilization of addiction-specific services averaged about 2 inpatient admissions per 1,000 members per year, with an average length of stay of 10 days, and an average of 74 outpatient visits per 1,000 members per year. These utilization levels were similar to levels found in previous HMO surveys.

The Influence of Cost-Containment Systems on Patient Care

A recent study by the General Accounting Office examined the effect of network-based managed care health plans on health care costs (General Accounting Office 1993). In 1992, enrollment in managed care plans using provider networks accounted for more than half of all employees covered by employer group health insurance. This proportion grew from 5% in 1980 to 55% in 1992. Overall, the results of the study gave little evidence that such networks resulted in major cost saving when the data were corrected for age and health of participants. Both network-based managed care and managed indemnity plans (accounting for about 41% of covered employees) experienced similar rates of premium growth over the previous 6 years. The GAO report, however, did not focus on mental health or substance use disorders treatment.

Several studies have investigated the impact of managed care systems on addiction treatment. N. A. Miller (1992) examined access to care and continuity and quality of treatment for 243 county government employees referred for addiction treatment by an employee assistance program (EAP). About half of those employees were covered by a fee-for-service plan, 38% were enrolled in HMOs, and 14% belonged to IPAs. Miller found decreased access to care in the IPAs and network-based HMOs. Access was also negatively correlated with co-payments and treatment limits in all systems. Treatment progress ratings were lower in staff model HMOs and were also negatively correlated with limits on benefits. The presence of addiction specialists on staff, ongoing professional development, and coordinated care were in turn associated with both better access to and progress in treatment.

Ellis (1992) traced drug (other than alcohol or nicotine) treatment costs incurred by one large private employer before and after a major change in insurance coverage offered by the company. The new benefit system included the use of case management and a PPO for all mental health and addiction treatment. The plan covered about 140,000 individuals. During the 2 years before the change, more than 90% of the cost of drug treatment was spent for inpatient care; after the change, the total dollars spent on drug treatment deceased precipitously—by 62% the first year and 39% the second year. Also following the change in the company's health care system, the cost of inpatient care contributed proportionally less to the total expenditure for health care, but the cost of outpatient and office visits also fell slightly. About half of the reduction was attributable to fewer patients receiving treatment (about one-third fewer treatment episodes per patient) and the rest was attributable to lower cost per treatment episode. Prior to the new system being instituted, 40% of patients treated for drug dependence in a year also received treatment in the following year. This proportion decreased to 25% after the restructuring. Ellis (1992) documented a drastic decrease in the amount of treatment for drug dependence provided, with a large consequent saving for the employer. The impact on individual patients and their families was not measured. Whether some of these patients shifted the locus of their care to the public treatment system or whether they were treated under other diagnoses in medical or psychiatric services was also not studied. Finally, the patients' treatment outcomes were not measured. Whether or not these findings can be generalized to other employers is also not clear, because the employer studied had a much higher than average addiction treatment cost before the change in the benefit system.

Looking at its own experience in providing consultation services to more than 2,000 private employers, Hewitt Associates estimated that the addition of a case management system with a utilization review plan that monitors all mental health and addiction treatment would save the average employer 5%–10% of the costs of an indemnity plan (McArdle et al. 1993). Hewitt further estimated that a plan that includes "a well-managed employee assistance program and utilization review with preferred discounting" (McArdle et al. 1993, p. 17) could reduce overall costs of mental health and addiction care by 25%–35% through decreasing inpatient costs by 30%–40% and outpatient costs by 10%–20%.

A study of McDonnell Douglas's cost savings through the use of an EAP to oversee the care of employees treated for mental and substance use disorders ("McDonnell Douglas Corporation's EAP Produces Hard Data" 1989) compared employees who received addiction treatment with EAP involvement to employees who received treatment independent of the company's EAP. In addition, a matched control group of employees with no addiction treatment history was used for comparison. All groups were tracked for a 6-year period (3 years before treatment and 3 years after treatment). Although both EAP and non-EAP groups showed improvement, the EAP group showed much greater decreases in absenteeism (44% fewer days), job loss (81% fewer terminations), and total medical costs, as well as decreases in costs attributable to their addictive disorder. Posttreatment family medical costs were also significantly lower for the EAP group. The results from the study indicated that the EAP had a positive effect on structuring addiction treatment.

An additional finding in the McDonnell Douglas study concerned HMO-based treatment. Approximately half of the EAP clients followed were enrolled in HMOs. Because claims data were not available from these providers, no comparative cost savings analysis was possible, but the outcome measures of absenteeism (days lost) and turnover rates (jobs lost) were measured. Although the absenteeism rate was comparable between HMO and fee-for-services patients during the first year after treatment, absenteeism rates were substantially higher in the HMO group during subsequent years. In addition, attrition rates were much higher. An HMO patient was 3 times more likely to lose his or her job than a patient in fee-for-service treatment. These differences were not explainable by demographic differences or by variations in the initial severity of illness (Smith and Mahoney 1989).

The findings discussed above point out the urgent need to gain additional knowledge about the effects on treatment outcome of different health care delivery systems. From the few studies reported so far, it seems that care management systems may either enhance or reduce treatment effectiveness, depending on how the systems are structured and implemented.

Medicare

Medicare is a federally financed and administered health insurance program that covers about 32 million Americans (Gerstein and Harwood 1990), mostly elderly people and a smaller number of disabled individuals under age 65 years. More than 95% of Americans over age 65 years and about 1.2% of Americans under age 65 years receive Medicare coverage. Although the younger disabled group accounts for far fewer enrollees than the older group, they are disproportionately represented in Medicare costs for addiction treatment (C. Lubinsky, National Council on Alcoholism and Drug Dependence, personal communication, 1993).

Medicare has two parts: Part A reimburses for hospital care and Part B reimburses physician fees. Until 1983, hospital inpatient services were paid on a cost-based retrospective reimbursement basis. At that time, a prospective payment system was introduced, using diagnosis-related groups (DRGs) as a basis for payment. The DRGs proposed for addiction treatment at that time did not distinguish between admissions for detoxification only and those for intensive inpatient rehabilitative treatment, creating a system divorced from clinical reality. After receiving considerable protest from clinicians, administrators, and field organizations (e.g., the National Council on Alcoholism and Drug Dependence [NCADD]), the Health Care Financing Administration (HCFA) withdrew these DRGs for restudy. In 1985, a new set of DRGs relating to the treatment of substance use disorders was introduced. In 1987, they were implemented in all hospitals. The current DRGs distinguish between admissions for detoxification and those for additional intensive inpatient care. However, they do not distinguish between the types of psychoactive substance disorders, nor do they recognize differences in treatment needs based on age, severity of dependence, dependence on multiple substances, social stability, or level of deterioration (Institute of Medicine 1990). (Problems with DRGs are not limited to Medicare, as other payers have also adopted the Medicare prospective payment system.)

A particularly difficult problem for the addiction treatment field is the limitation of Medicare coverage to hospital-based treatment. Freestanding residential facilities are not covered, even though they may offer similar services to inpatient hospital-based units at a lower cost. In addition, Medicare Part A imposes a 190-day lifetime limit on hospital days for psychiatric care (including addiction treatment), a limit not imposed on general medical care admissions.

Medicare Part B also has considerable limitations: it covers outpatient care in medically based settings only and requires a 50% co-payment. Medicare classifies addiction treatment as a subset of psychiatric care and subjects such treatment to the same limits. The recent institution of a new Medicare fee schedule has created a special problem for psychiatrists, including those treating addictive disorders. The Omnibus Budget Reconciliation Act of 1989 mandated the development of this new schedule, which was to be based on the relative values of work and resources used by physicians in providing services and to be used to replace the previous fee schedule based on usual and customary fees. This resource-based relative value scale (RBRVS) system was gradually implemented beginning January 1, 1992. Part of the rationale for the change in fee structure was the application of a more equitable method to balance cognitive physician work (e.g., consultation, examination, diagnosis, prescription) against work related to performing procedures. However, the system has been criticized for unfairness in many respects (American Psychiatric Association 1993a; Maloney 1992). Some of these failings particularly affect psychiatrists. For example, the downward adjustment of relative value units of payment to maintain budget neutrality in the adoption of RBRVS penalizes psychiatrists and other specialties with higher proportions of cognitive work. In addition, HCFA's value performance standards (assumptions that physicians will increase their volume or intensity of services to compensate for losses in reimbursement) affect psychiatrists disproportionately because they are not able to make such adjustments (American Psychiatric Association 1993a).

It is also notable that the initial clinical materials used to develop the time and resource psychiatric RBRVS work standards did not include case examples of the evaluation and treatment of substance use disorders. These case examples were added later, only after objections from psychiatrists providing addiction treatment. As in the case of the Medicare inpatient reimbursement methodology, the implications of this physician payment system are far wider than the Medicare system itself: other insurers model their reimbursement structures on the Medicare system.

An additional problem for addiction psychiatry is the prohibition that forbids patient payment of discrepancies between Medicare reimbursement and physicians' fees. This restriction limits the willingness of many physicians to accept Medicare patients. It therefore limits access to and choice of a psychiatrist for retirees (including retired physicians) and chronically disabled patients.

Although a precise estimate for the total amount of Medicare expenditure attributed to addictive disorders treatment is not available, Adams et al. (1993) did identify all alcohol-related hospitalizations nationwide for Medicare recipients over age 65 years. For the year 1989, the overall rate of such hospital admissions was 48.2 per 10,000 of the elderly population (54.7 for men and 14.8 for women). This represented 1.1% of all hospitalizations for those age 65 years and older, or more than 87,000 admissions.

In 29% of these, an alcohol-related diagnosis was the primary diagnosis listed. These 33,000 admissions alone accounted for Medicare Part A expenditures of more than $233.5 million. They included treatment for both alcohol abuse-dependence and alcohol-related complications. It has been roughly estimated that in 1990 $700 million was spent for all alcohol and other drug treatment covered in both Parts A and B of Medicare (M. Belfer, Substance Abuse and Mental Health Services Administration, personal communication, May 1993).

Medicaid

Medicaid is a health insurance program jointly financed by federal and state funds under Title XIX of the Social Security Act, the purpose of which is to provide medical services to needy individuals. Each state administers its own program—including setting eligibility requirements, reimbursement rates, and types and amounts of services covered—within federally set guidelines. These mandates include covering all individuals receiving federally assisted welfare or disability benefits and providing a basic set of core medical services (e.g., inpatient and outpatient hospital care, prenatal care, preventive care for children) ("New Research Studies Show" 1993). In addition to the mandated services, 32 optional services for which federal matching funds are provided may be included in the plan. This list includes outpatient treatment for psychoactive substance use disorders. The federal contribution to state Medicaid costs varies from 50% to 80%, based on the per capita income of the state. States may also add to their plans services for which federal funds are not provided.

Some Medicaid coverage restrictions cause particular problems for addiction treatment. One of these restrictions is the prohibition of federally participating Medicaid coverage for any services in so-called institutions for mental disorders (IMDs) for individuals between ages 22 years and 65 years. These IMDs include both psychiatric hospitals and freestanding inpatient addiction treatment units. This limits the access of Medicaid-insured adults to inpatient intensive treatment and to most specialized dual diagnosis inpatient units.

Surveys of Medicaid programs in different states reveal wide disparities in the extent to which addictive disorder treatment is included (Institute of Medicine 1990; "New Research Studies Show" 1993). Although Medicaid is not a major funding source for addiction services as a whole, it is so for some states (e.g., New York) (Institute of Medicine 1990). Relatively few studies of Medicaid addiction treatment utilization have been reported. One survey in the state of Washington found that, although patients with a diagnosis of drug (other than alcohol) dependence were a small proportion of the total Medicaid caseload, they consumed a 37% greater than average amount of resources ($5,789/year for addicted patients in fiscal year 1990 versus $2,128 for all other recipients). Drug dependence treatment itself accounted for only 4% of total Medicaid costs (National Association of State Alcohol and Abuse Directors, undated).

Another recent study by the Center on Addiction and Substance Abuse (1993) included estimates of the total impact of addictive disorders on Medicaid hospital costs nationwide. It was found that, of the total $21.6 billion spent by Medicaid on inpatient hospital care in 1991, $700,000 (about 3%) was devoted to the care of substance use disorders (e.g., substance abuse-dependence, psychosis, delirium). However, Medicaid spent $4.2 billion, or 19% of the total, on hospital stays for the more than 70 diagnoses attributable in whole or part to the excessive use of psychoactive substances (including tobacco). Projections for the year 1994 are that, of total Medicaid inpatient costs of $146 billion, 28% or $41 billion will be attributable to substance-related medical conditions.

The 1990 Institute of Medicine study by Gerstein and Harwood identified Medicaid as an underutilized resource for the support of addiction treatment. However, many states do not elect to include this coverage because of concerns for growing costs. Various states have implemented Medicaid cost control systems. The Oregon experiment is discussed in the section "The Effectiveness and Cost-Benefit of Addiction Treatment," above. Other states have adopted HMO systems for Medicaid recipients. A Pennsylvania experiment, begun in 1986, established a combination of an HMO type system and fee-for-service addiction treatment (Duggar 1991). Preliminary results of an evaluation of this project found that system problems and constraints had interfered with its utilization reduction and cost-saving goals.

Although precise estimates are not available, it is believed that at least $1 billion was spent by Medicaid on specialty treatment for substance use disorders in 1990 (M. Belfer, Substance Abuse and Mental Health Services Administration, personal communication, May 1993).

Civilian Health and Medical Program
of the Uniformed Services

The Civilian Health and Medical Program of the Uniformed Services
(CHAMPUS) is a health care reimbursement system funded through the
Department of Defense that pays for services provided to military retirees
and the dependents of active duty, deceased, and retired military personnel
when they receive care in civilian hospitals and by other nonmilitary
providers. In 1991, the General Accounting Office reviewed current
CHAMPUS benefits for mental health and addiction treatment. As of
October 1, 1991, acute inpatient care for mental illness or drug dependence
was provided for 30 days/year for adults and 45 days/year for patients
under age 19 years. Residential treatment was limited to 150 days/year. For
alcohol abuse-dependence, CHAMPUS covered up to 7 days/year of inpatient detoxification. Inpatient rehabilitation was limited to a single 21-day
stay annually, with a lifetime limit of three inpatient stays. A special
waiver of these limits may be obtained in some cases (General Accounting
Office 1991). Outpatient visits were limited to 60 visits/year for alcoholism
treatment and 104 for treatment of other drug dependence (the same limit
as mental health). Co-payments were 20% for dependents of active duty
personnel and 25% for all others. These benefits compared favorably with
those provided in private industry and to federal employees. Annual deductibles of $150/person and $300/family were applied to all medical
outpatient services and were not specific for mental health or addiction
treatment.

Addiction treatment inpatient admissions reimbursed by the CHAM-
PUS system for fiscal year 1991 totaled nearly 5,600. Of these, the vast
majority of admissions were for the diagnosis of alcohol dependence
($n = 2,579$), with cocaine dependence ($n = 422$), alcohol intoxication
($n = 390$), alcohol abuse ($n = 387$), drug dependence ($n = 322$), drug abuse
($n = 296$), and alcoholic psychosis ($n = 203$) also contributing significantly
to the total. Of a total cost of about $34.5 million, the treatment for alcohol
abuse-dependence diagnoses contributed $16.7 million, and cocaine
abuse-dependence contributed $3.4 million (J. E. Tart, Office of the Assis-
tant Secretary of Defense, personal communication, December 1992).
Estimates for total CHAMPUS expenditures for outpatient addiction treatment are not currently available. However, based on the experience of

previous years, inpatient care makes up the vast majority of the total annual cost of treatment.

Direct Public Support

Federal Support

As summarized in the first section of this chapter, the federal role in supporting addiction treatment services includes funding from the budgets of many agencies. In some cases (e.g., Medicare, Medicaid, CHAMPUS), these funds are paid to providers as insurance reimbursement. In this section we describe the major sources of direct federal support for treatment services—through the alcohol and drug block grants to the states, direct program grants, and support of treatment provided by various branches of the military and by the Department of Veterans Affairs and the Indian Health Service.

Block grants. In 1981, funds granted by the various Alcohol, Drug Abuse and Mental Health Administration (ADAMHA) agencies to support alcoholism and other drug treatment programs (federal formula grants and direct program grants) were consolidated into a newly named *federal block grant.* At the time this change was made, there was also a transfer of total responsibility for the management of these funds to the states, and a decrease in overall funding of 25% (Besteman 1992). Additional funds were appropriated for the block grants by the Congress in 1986, the first increase in block grant funding since the mid-1970s. At that time, Congress also required that specified proportions of the block grant funds be set aside for particular purposes (e.g., to improve programming for women). These and other later set-asides and restrictions restored some federal control over how the block grant was spent.

With the reorganization of the ADAMHA agencies in 1992, the responsibility for the block grant remained with the former Office of Treatment Improvement, now named the Center for Substance Abuse Treatment (CSAT), part of the newly formed Substance Abuse and Mental Health Services Administration.

For federal fiscal year 1994, the Congress appropriated $1.17 billion for the alcohol and drug block grant ("Hike Approved for Block Grant" 1992). These funds are administered by the states to support both treatment and prevention programs ("Federal Block Grant Regulations Issued" 1993). Regulations for the use of these funds include the following:

✦ At least 35% of the grant must be spent on alcohol services and 35% on drug services; the remainder may be used for either at state discretion.
✦ Funded treatment agencies must provide continuing education to their staff.
✦ At least 5% of funded agencies must undergo quality review by the state.
✦ At least 20% of the grant must be spent on services for at-risk populations not currently in need of treatment services.
✦ At least 5% of funds must be set aside for increasing the availability of services for pregnant women and women with dependent children. Pregnant women in need of treatment must be given admission priority.
✦ At least 2% of the grant must be used for early intervention and prevention of AIDS.
✦ States must provide treatment services for tuberculosis.
✦ States must ensure confidentiality of records.
✦ Up to 3% of the grant is set aside for providing technical assistance, data collection, and program evaluation.

Direct federal grant support.   In addition to the block grants, CSAT administers several programs awarding direct grants to treatment providers. These grants encourage the development of new models of treatment for underserved populations as well as serve other specific needs. For federal fiscal year 1993, $133.9 million was appropriated for treatment improvement grants ("Hike Approved for Block Grant" 1992). These projects are funded in part by federal drug asset forfeiture funds (i.e., assets seized from individuals arrested for drug-related crimes). Among directly funded program categories are the following:

✦ Community partnership grants
✦ Capacity expansion grants
✦ Residential treatment for women and their children
✦ Residential treatment for pregnant and postpartum women
✦ Model comprehensive treatment for critical populations

✦ Cooperative agreements for addiction and recovery systems in target cities
✦ Substance abuse treatment in state and local criminal justice systems
✦ Capitol area demonstration program (applies to Washington, D.C.)

Department of Veterans Affairs. The Department of Veterans Affairs (VA) is one of the largest providers of treatment for the psychoactive substance use disorders in the world.

For federal fiscal year 1991, the VA sponsored formal addiction treatment in all of its 153 medical centers and freestanding outpatient clinics, with an additional 13 detoxification programs (Moos et al. 1992). The VA also provides care through contracts with community-based halfway houses. Of the 553,236 patients discharged from all VA medical centers in 1991, 25.4% ($n = 140,550$) had a primary or secondary diagnosis of a substance use disorder. Of these, 49,899 received care in addiction treatment units, representing 35.5% of the discharges with substance use disorder diagnoses, with 21% being treated in psychiatric units only and 43.5%, in medical-surgical units only. In addition, 11,322 (29.9%) of the veterans discharged from VA extended care facilities had a primary or secondary diagnosis of addictive disorder.

Of the patients treated in specialized inpatient addiction units, 48% had a diagnosis of alcohol dependence; 12%, other drug dependence; and 41%, both. Nearly 28% had an additional psychiatric diagnosis.

At least 7.5% of all VA outpatients ($n = 184,631$) were treated for substance use disorders in 1991. These patients accounted for 16% of all outpatient visits. In addition, 86,000 family members or significant others were seen in conjunction with the addicted patients. Furthermore, approximately 6,000 patients were placed in VA-contracted addiction program halfway houses (R. T. Suchinsky, Department of Veterans Affairs, personal communication, December 1992).

Costs for this care include $519 million for addiction-specific inpatient services, $835 million for outpatient services, and $8.5 million for halfway house care, for a total of $1.36 billion.

Support by the U. S. military. National studies of the addiction treatment system generally survey only civilian programs, yet the U. S. military services employ about 1,774,000 active duty personnel. These personnel are divided between the services as follows: Army, 31%; Navy, 30%; Marine Corps, 11%; and Air Force, 29% (Bray et al. 1992). Because this military workforce is 85% male, with 66.4% of those being between ages 21 years and 34 years, it constitutes a group that is demographically at high risk for psychoactive substance use disorders. In 1992, a survey of more than 16,000 active duty military personnel worldwide was prepared for the Department of Defense (Bray et al. 1992). Heavy alcohol use (5 or more drinks per occasion at least once a week) was reported by 15.2% of the respondents. Productivity loss because of alcohol use was reported by 16.4%, serious consequences from alcohol use by 7.6%, and alcohol dependence symptoms by 5.2%. Illicit drug use was reported by 6.2% during the preceding year and 3.4% during the preceding 30 days. Serious consequences from drug use were reported by 0.4% and dependence symptoms by 0.7%. Current cigarette smoking was reported by 35% and heavy smoking (one or more packs per day) by 18%. Although these levels represented significant declines from similar surveys over the previous 13 years, the need for addiction treatment services persists in the military.

Three branches of the military operate their own prevention and treatment facilities; the Navy program also treats members of the Marine Corps. The Army operates an Alcohol and Drug Prevention and Abuse Control Program within each of its approximately 120 installations worldwide. These programs provide outpatient counseling and urine testing. Patients in need of residential care are referred to one of eight inpatient programs that provide detoxification and receive 6–8 weeks of intensive inpatient rehabilitation. Inpatient treatment is followed by a year of outpatient counseling after the patient's return to duty. Army facilities also counsel dependents, including adolescents.

The Air Force operates 9 inpatient treatment units worldwide, the largest of which has 23 beds. These units offer similar services to those of the Army programs, and are also followed by outpatient counseling (Department of Defense, personal communication, 1992).

The Navy program includes 4 large alcohol rehabilitation centers, 19 smaller alcohol rehabilitation departments in naval medical centers, and 80 counseling and assistance centers located in local commands. The centers provide assessment, referral, counseling, and follow-up for those treated in inpatient settings (R. E. Bally, Department of Defense, personal communication, December 1992). Navy inpatient alcohol-drug programs treated approximately 6,500 patients in fiscal year 1992 (about 4,000 Navy personnel, 1,400 Marine Corps personnel, and 1,000 others). Outpatient programs conducted nearly 20,000 alcohol and drug screenings and counseled about 3,000 patients (2,750 Navy, 120 Marine, and 120 other) (R. E. Bally, Department of Defense, personal communication, December 1992). Cost-benefit studies of the Navy program, summarized in the section "The Effectiveness and Cost-Benefit of Addiction Treatment," above, have demonstrated considerable cost savings. Parallel studies for the other services are not available.

Indian Health Service. Among Native American Indians and Alaskan Natives, substance use disorders are recognized as major health problems. As part of its program of health services to these populations, the Indian Health Service provides addiction treatment. The White House's Office of National Drug Control Policy identified approximately $35.3 million spent for these alcohol and other drug treatment services in 1991. Indian Health Services include alcohol and drug prevention services, fetal alcohol syndrome prevention services, and adolescent services as well as treatment and aftercare at eight regional centers. The sum spent on addiction services in 1991 represented about 2% of the total agency's total budget (Office of the National Drug Control Policy 1992).

State and Local Support

As discussed in the section "Financing of the Addiction Treatment System," above, the proportion of public financing provided by state and local governments to community-based programs grew during the 1980s to surpass the proportion funded by the federal government. The State Alcohol and Drug Abuse Profile for the fiscal year 1991 (Butynski et al. 1992) identified $3.2 billion in support for prevention and treatment programs that received at least some state-administered funds. Of that total, 29.2% came from the federal block grants and 8.5% from other federal programs. Of the remaining 62%, 47% was derived from state and local funding (34.4% from state alcohol and drug agency funds, 5.2% from other state agencies, and 6.9% from local or county agencies) and 15.5% came from other sources. About 75% of the total was expended on treatment. The 1991 NDATUS survey identified approximately $1.4 billion of state and local support, or about 34% of the $4.14 billion expended on treatment services nationwide (Substance Abuse and Mental Health Services Administration 1992).

Other Sources of Support

Charitable Contributions and Foundations

There is no single source available to track the amount of financial support provided to the addiction treatment system by foundations, charities, and corporations. The majority of community-based, nonprofit treatment programs conduct some fund-raising activities independently, through the local United Way program, or both. Churches provide support for some programs as do the Salvation Army and other national charitable organizations.

Private foundations are also contributors to the support of selected treatment programs. A 1989 study by the Foundation Center examined overall giving for alcohol and drug-related purposes by more than 450 foundations between 1981 and 1987. The total of reported grants grew from $4.36 million in 1980 to $26.36 million in 1987. Of the $87 million granted during this 8-year period, $41.8 million represented grants to treatment agencies. For the year 1987, about $9.9 million were granted to treatment programs. Although the total funds devoted to alcohol- and drug-related purposes was considerable, as a proportion of total giving by the foundations reported in the study, the amount was small, and in fact represented only 1% of the grants awarded in 1987. Most of the funds granted for treatment went to hospitals, rehabilitation centers, and residential communities, with smaller amounts to outpatient and other services. Priority was given to services for adolescents, with women's services the second most common type of program to receive support. Since the Foundation Center report was written, several large foundations, most notably the Robert Wood Johnson Foundation, have become involved in granting funds to support community responses to substance use-related problems. However, there is still a great deal of potential foundation support that might be tapped in the future.

Asset Seizure

Both federal and state laws allow the seizure and forfeiture of assets used in the illicit drug trade. These assets are in turn used by the appropriate unit of government to help fund antidrug activities. Seized assets characteristically include both cash and property (e.g., automobiles, buildings, aircraft). Property may be sold and the proceeds deposited in a special fund. Most of the forfeited assets are used to support law enforcement activities, but some funds, buildings, and other properties have been made available to nonprofit community prevention and treatment programs.

At the federal level, the Comprehensive Crime Control Act of 1984 established the Assets Forfeiture Fund within the Department of Justice (Office of National Drug Control Policy 1992a). According to the White House's National Drug Strategy report, nearly $630 million in cash and property was obtained in 1991 under federal asset forfeiture laws (Office of National Drug Control Policy 1992b). Some of these assets were shared with state and local agencies, whereas others were used to fund various programs related to the "war on drugs." For the fiscal year 1993, two treatment grant programs funded through the Substance Abuse and Mental Health Services Administration—the Capacity Expansion Program and the Residential Treatment for Mothers and Children Program—were scheduled to receive $15.3 million and $5 million, respectively ("Hike Approved for Block Grant" 1992). Asset forfeiture promises to be a continuing source of nontax funding of antidrug activities. An increase in the proportion of asset forfeiture funds spent on treatment could improve the ability of federal, state, and local jurisdictions to support treatment services.

Dedicated Taxes

Over many years, proposals have been made at both the federal and state levels to impose special taxes on alcoholic beverages, tobacco products, or both, with the proceeds being dedicated to the support of prevention, research, or treatment. The theory of such taxes is simple. If excessive use of a product creates costs to society, in particular to government, users of the product should pay these costs in proportion to their use (Manning et al. 1991). Proponents of dedicated taxes point to gasoline taxes used for road construction and maintenance as a model of fairness. They argue that additional resources for treatment can be raised without increasing the tax burden on the general public because 50% of the alcoholic beverages sold in the United States is consumed by 5% of the total population (Moore and Gerstein 1981). They also point out that increasing the price of a product decreases overall consumption, especially by adolescents.

Opponents of dedicated taxes argue that governments would simply deduct a similar amount of general fund support for treatment to make up for the funds raised by a dedicated tax. They also point out that linking a treatment or research budget to sales of alcohol or tobacco would result in an interest in maintaining or increasing sales of the product. Legislatures and executive branches of government generally dislike dedicated taxes because they limit government's discretion in the use of tax funds. Although there have been several increases in cigarette and alcohol taxes at both federal and state levels in recent years, in most cases these revenues have gone into the general fund of the jurisdiction. Recent health care reform proposals have linked increased taxes on tobacco and alcohol to the funding of health care.

Funding of Clinical Research

Although the proportion of the overall network of treatment services funded as part of a clinical research project is very small, these programs play an important role in the advancement of practical knowledge about substance use disorders and their treatment. An example of such a facility is the Clinical Research Center at the New York Research Institute on Addiction in Buffalo, New York.

Several investigators studying the levels of support for research on mental illness and addictive disorders have concluded that these areas of research are underfunded, both in relation to the number of individuals affected by the illness and to levels of social cost (Institute of Medicine 1980).

A 1992 review by Pincus and Fine (1992) found that mental illness and alcohol and drug research combined represented only 4.7% of all health research support, but mental illness and substance use disorders accounted for 12% of the total societal health cost for the same survey period. Of the total societal health cost, 3.4% is devoted to research, but the proportion devoted to research on mental health and addictive disorders is much lower—only 1.3%. The economic consequences of mental illness, alcoholism, and other drug dependence are comparable with those of heart disease and cancer, yet the federal government's research funding for mental illness is less than 45% of its research commitment to the National Cancer Institute and barely 75% of its research commitment to heart disease. In 1988, approximately $859 million was spent on all alcohol, other drug (exclusive of tobacco), and mental health research. Of this total, 64% was funded by the three federal institutes—National Institute of Mental Health (NIMH), NIDA, and NIAAA; 7.5%, by other federal agencies (including 2% by the VA); 8%, by state funding; 17%, by pharmaceutical companies and hospitals; and 3.5%, by foundations.

In addition, compared with general health research, alcohol, drug, and mental health research derives a smaller proportion of support from private industry and voluntary health organizations and foundations, leaving a greater reliance on the federal government. Funding from the National Institutes of Health in 1988 (before the transfer of NIMH, NIDA, and NIAAA to NIH) accounted for 34% of general health research expenditures, but NIMH, NIDA, and NIAAA funding represent 64% of research support for mental health and addictive disorders. Although private industry provided 44% of all health research, it provided only 17% of research in mental health and addiction. Virtually none of this industry support was devoted to alcohol and drug research.

The federally launched "Decade of the Brain" may present a window of opportunity in advocating for addictive disorder research. The search for better chemical treatments for addictive disorders has led to the establishment of the Medications Development Divisions within NIDA and NIAAA. Psychiatrists can play a major role in educating funding agencies and the public about the psychobiology of substance use disorders, particularly new discoveries in brain-behavior relationships. Psychiatrists can engage in direct research or advocate for its support. They can also help disseminate results of research findings, especially those concerning treatment outcome and resource utilization (American Psychiatric Association 1993b; College on Problems of Drug Dependence 1993). Basic and clinical research are society's most promising long-term strategies for reducing the prevalence and societal cost of addictive disorders and for improving the effectiveness of treatment.

References

Adams WL, Yuan Z, Barboriak JJ, et al: Alcohol-related hospitalizations of elderly people: prevalence and geographic variation in the United States. JAMA 270:1222–1225, 1993

American Medical Association: Factors Contributing to the Health Care Cost Problem. Chicago, IL, American Medical Association, 1993

American Psychiatric Association, Division of Government Relations: Resource-Based Relative Value Scale (RBRVS) Medicare Fee Schedule. Washington, DC, American Psychiatric Association, 1993a

American Psychiatric Association, Division of Government Relations: Mental Illness, Alcoholism, and Substance Abuse: A Recommendation for the FY 1994 Appropriation for the National Institute of Mental Health, National Institute on Alcohol Abuse and Alcoholism, and National Institute on Drug Abuse. Washington, DC, American Psychiatric Association, 1993b

Barr HL, Ottenberg DJ, Rosen A: Mortality of treated alcoholics and drug addicts: the benefits of abstinence. J Stud Alcohol 45:440–452, 1984

Besteman KJ: Federal leadership in building the national drug treatment system, in Extent and Adequacy of Insurance Coverage for Substance Abuse Services (Drug Abuse Services Research Series, Vol 2; DHHS Publ No ADM-92-1998). Washington, DC, US Government Printing Office, 1992

Hike approved for block grant: most programs get more money. Alcoholism and Drug Abuse Weekly 4:1–2, 1992

Blose JO, Holder HD: The utilization of medical care by treated alcoholics: longitudinal patterns by age, gender and type of care. J Subst Abuse 3:13–27, 1991

Borthwick RB: Summary of cost-benefit study results for navy alcoholism rehabilitation programs. Navy Alcohol Prevention Program, Technical Report No. 346. Washington, DC, US Government Printing Office, 1977

Bray RM, Kroutil LA, Luckey JW, et al (eds): Highlights of 1992 worldwide survey of substance abuse and health behaviors among military personnel (RTI/232U/5154/06-02DR). Washington, DC, Office of Assistant Secretary for Defense (Health Affairs), November 6, 1992

Bullick KD, Reed RJ, Grant I: Reduced mortality risk in alcoholics who achieve long-term abstinence. JAMA 267:668–672, 1992

Bureau of Labor Statistics: Employee Benefits in State and Local Governments, 1987 (Bureau of Labor Statistics Bulletin 2309). Washington, DC, US Department of Labor, 1987

Butinsky W, Reda JL, Bartosch W, et al: State resources and services related to alcohol and other drug abuse problems, fiscal year 1991: an analysis of state alcohol and drug abuse profile data. Washington, DC, National Association of State Alcohol and Drug Abuse Directors, 1991

Butynski W, Reda JL, Bartosch W, et al: State resources and services related to alcohol and other drug abuse problems, fiscal year 1991: a report for the Office of Applied Studies, Substance Abuse and Mental Health Services Administration. Washington, DC, National Association of State Alcohol and Drug Abuse Directors, 1992

Caliber Associates (eds): Cost Benefit Study of the Navy's Level III Alcohol Rehabilitation Program Phase Two: Rehabilitation Versus Replacement Costs, 1989

Cartwright WS, Kaple JM: Introduction and summary, in Economic Costs, Cost-Effectiveness, Financing and Community-Based Drug Treatment. National Institute on Drug Abuse Research Monograph No 113 (DHHS Publ No ADM-91-1823). Edited by Cartwright WS, Kaple JM. Washington, DC, US Government Printing Office, 1991a, pp 1–9

Cartwright WS, Kaple JM (eds): Economic Costs, Cost-Effectiveness, Financing, and Community-Based Drug Treatment. National Institute on Drug Abuse Research Monograph No 113 (DHHS Publ No ADM-91-1823). Washington, DC, US Government Printing Office, 1991b

Center on Addiction and Substance Abuse: The cost of substance abuse to America's health care system report 1, Medicaid hospital costs: a CASA report. New York, Center on Addiction and Substance Abuse at Columbia University, 1993

College on Problems of Drug Dependence: Role of the federal government in drug abuse control: research needs. Position paper sent to President Clinton, January 1993

Davis K, Anderson G, Rowland D, et al: Health Care Cost Containment. Baltimore, MD, Johns Hopkins University Press, 1990

Department of Justice: What are the costs to society of illegal drug abuse? in Drugs, Crime and the Justice System. A National Report From the Bureau of Justice Statistics (NCJ-133652). Washington, DC, US Government Printing Office, 1992, pp 126–127

Duggar BC: Community-based drug treatment reimbursement: progress and barriers, in Economic Costs, Cost-Effectiveness, Financing, and Community-Based Drug Treatment. Edited by Cartwright WS, Kaple JM. NIDA Research Monograph 113, 1991, pp 148–164

Ellis RP: Drug abuse treatment patterns before and after managed care. NIDA Drug Abuse Services Research Series. Washington, DC, April 1992

Emrick CD: A review of psychologically oriented treatment of alcoholism, II: the relative effectiveness of different treatment approaches and the effectiveness of treatment versus no treatment. J Stud Alcohol 36:88–108, 1975

Federal block grant regulations issued by CSAT. Alcoholism Report 4:2–6, 1993

Filstead W: Treatment Outcome: An Evaluation of Adult Residential Treatment Services. Parkside Medical Services Corporation, Park Ridge, IL, January 1989a

Filstead W: Treatment Outcome: An Evaluation of Youth Residential Treatment Services. Parkside Medical Services Corporation, Park Ridge, IL, January 1989b

Finney JW, Moos RH: Matching patients to treatments: conceptual and methodological issues. J Stud Alcohol 47:122–134, 1986

Finney JW, Moos RH: The long-term course of treated alcoholism, II: predictors and correlates of 10-year functioning and mortality. J Stud Alcohol 53:142–153, 1992

Ford MQ: The incredible shrinking utilization: report of a MEDSTAT study. National Association of Addiction Treatment Providers Review 13:2–5, 1992

Foundation Center: Alcohol and Drug Abuse Funding: An Analysis of Foundation Grants. A Study by The Foundation Center. New York, Foundation Center, 1989

General Accounting Office: Defense health care: CHAMPUS mental health benefits greater than those under other health plans. Report to the Chairman, Subcommittee on Military Personnel and Compensation, Committee on Armed Services, House of Representatives (Report No GAO/HRD-92-20). Washington, DC, General Accounting Office, 1991

General Accounting Office: Utilization review: information on external review organizations. Fact sheet for the Chairman, Select Committee on Aging, House of Representatives (Report No GAO/HRD-93-22FS). Washington, DC, General Accounting Office, 1992

General Accounting Office: Managed health care effect on employers' costs difficult to measure (Report No GAO/HRD 94.3). Washington, DC, General Accounting Office, 1993

Gerstein DR, Harwood HJ (eds): Treating Drug Problems, Vol 1. Washington, DC, National Academy Press, 1990

Gibbs L, Flanagan J: Prognostic indicators of alcoholism treatment outcome. Int J Addict 12:1097–1141, 1977

Glaser FB: Anybody got a match? treatment research and the matching hypothesis, in Alcoholism Treatment in Transition. Edited by Edwards G, Grant M. London, Croom Helm, 1980, pp 178–196

Gottheil E, McLellan T, Druley K: Length of stay, patient severity and treatment outcome: sample data from the field of alcoholism. J Stud Alcohol 53:69–75, 1992

Harwood HJ, Napolitano DM, Kristiansen PL, et al: Economic costs to society of alcohol and drug abuse and mental illness: 1980. Report prepared for the Alcohol, Drug Abuse, and Mental Health Administration (RT1/2734/00-01FR). Research Triangle Park, NC, Research Triangle Institute, 1984

Harwood HJ, Thomson M, Nesmith T: Final Report: Healthcare Reform and Substance Abuse Treatment: The Cost of Financing Under Alternative Approaches. Fairfax, VA, Lewin-VHI, 1994

Hay/Huggins Company: Psychiatric benefits in employer-provided healthcare plans: 1992. Report prepared for National Association of Private Psychiatric Hospitals. Washington, DC, Hay/Huggins Company, 1992

Hayami DE, Freeborn DK: Effect of coverage on use of an HMO alcoholism treatment program, outcome, and medical care utilization. Am J Public Health 71:1133–1143, 1981

Health Insurance Association of America: 1992 Source Book of Health Insurance Data. Washington, DC, Health Insurance Association of America, 1993

Heien DM, Pittman DJ: The external costs of alcohol abuse. J Stud Alcohol 54:302–307, 1993

Hewitt Associates: Managing Health Care Costs. Lincolnshire, IL, Hewitt Associates, 1990

Hike approved for block grant: most programs get more money. Alcoholism and Drug Abuse Weekly 4:1–2, 1992

Hoffman NG, DeHart SS, Fulkerson JA: Medical care utilization as a function of recovery status following chemical addictions treatment. J Addict Dis 12:97–108, 1993

Hoffman NG, Miller NS: Treatment outcomes for abstinence-based programs. Psychiatric Annals 22:402–408, 1992

Hoffman NG, Halikas JA, Mee-Lee D, et al: Patient Placement Criteria for the Treatment of Psychoactive Substance Use Disorders. Washington, DC, American Society of Addiction Medicine, 1991

Holden C: Alcoholism and the medical cost crunch. Science 235:1132–1133, 1987

Holder HD, Blose JO: Alcoholism treatment and total health care utilization and costs. JAMA 256:1456–1460, 1986

Holder HD: Alcoholism treatment and potential health care cost saving. Med Care 25:52–71, 1987

Holder HD, Blose JO: The reduction of health care costs associated with alcoholism treatment: a 14-year longitudinal study. J Stud Alcohol 53:293–301, 1992

Horgan C, Marsden ME, Larson MJ, et al: Substance Abuse—The Nation's Number One Health Problem: Key Indicators for Policy. Waltham, MA, Institute for Health Policy, Brandeis University Press, 1993

Hubbard RL, Marsden ME, Rachal JV, et al. (eds): Drug Abuse Treatment: A National Study of Effectiveness. Chapel Hill, NC, University of North Carolina Press, 1989

Institute of Medicine: Alcoholism, Alcohol Abuse /and Related Problems: Opportunities for Research. Washington, DC, National Academy Press, 1980

Institute of Medicine: Prevention and Treatment of Alcohol Problems: Research Opportunities. Washington, DC, National Academy Press, 1989

Institute of Medicine: Broadening the Base of Treatment for Alcohol Problems. Washington, DC, American Psychiatric Press, 1990

Jones K, Vischi T: Impact of alcohol, drug abuse and mental health treatment on medical care utilization: a review of the research literature. Med Care 17 (suppl 12):1–82, 1979

Legal Action Center: Results of the Legal Action Center Insurance Benefit (Utilization Review) Study. Legal Action Center, 1992

Levin BL: Utilization and costs of substance abuse services within the HMO group. HMO Practice 7:28–34, 1993

Levin BL, Glasser JH: A national survey of prepaid mental health services. Hosp Community Psychiatry 35:350–355, 1984

Levin BL, Glasser JH, Jaffee CL Jr: National trends in coverage and utilization of mental health, alcohol, and substance abuse services within managed health care systems. Am J Public Health 78:1222–1223, 1988

Maloney JV: The resource-based relative value scale. JAMA 268:3363–3365, 1992

Manning WG, Keeler EB, Newhouse JP, et al (eds): The Costs of Poor Health Habits. Cambridge, MA, Harvard University Press, 1991

Macro International, Inc.: Managed care and substance abuse treatment: a need for dialogue (DHHS Publ No ADM 270-91-0007). Report to the Office for Treatment Improvement under Contract No ADM 270-91-007. Washington, DC, 1992

McArdle FB, Mahoney JJ, Yamamoto DH, et al: Testimony on mental health and substance abuse benefits and the Health Security Act of 1993 before the US Senate Committee on Labor and Human Resources, November 8, 1993

McDonnell Douglas Corporation's EAP produces hard data. The Almacan 19:18–26, 1989

McLellan AT, O'Brien CP, Metzger D, et al: How effective is substance abuse treatment—compared to what? in, Addictive States. Edited by O'Brien CP, Jaffe JH. New York, Raven, 1991, pp 231–252

McLellan AT, Grissom GR, Brill P, et al: Private substance abuse treatment: are some programs more effective than others? J Subst Abuse Treat 10:243–254, 1993

Miller J, Zeuschner A, Harwood HJ, et al (eds): Substance Abuse Treatment and Health Care Reform. Washington, DC, National Institute on Drug Abuse, 1993

Miller NA: An evaluation of substance misuse treatment providers used by an employee assistance program. Int J Addict 27(5):533–559, 1992

Moore MH, Gerstein DR (eds): Alcohol and Public Policy: Beyond the Shadow of Prohibition. Washington, DC, National Academy Press, 1981

Moos RH, Stephan M, Swindle R (eds): Health Services for VA Substance Abuse Patients: Utilization and Costs for Fiscal Year 1991. Department of Veterans Affairs, September 1992

National Association of Addiction Treatment Providers: Treatment is the answer: a white paper on the cost effectiveness of alcoholism and drug dependency treatment. Laguna Hills, CA, National Association of Addiction Treatment Providers, 1991

National Association of State Alcohol and Drug Abuse Directors: Survey on selected state alcohol and drug abuse agency's Medicaid funded services. Washington, DC, National Association of State Alcohol and Drug Abuse Directors (undated)

National Association of State Alcohol and Drug Abuse Directors: Treatment Works: The tragic cost of undervaluing treatment in the "drug war." Washington, DC, National Association of State Alcohol and Drug Abuse Directors, 1990

National Institute on Alcohol Abuse and Alcoholism: Estimating the Economic Cost of Alcohol Abuse. Alcohol Alert 11:PH 293, 1991

New research studies show costs and variability in Medicaid substance abuse programs. Connection 2:2–4, 1993

Office of National Drug Control Policy: 1992 National Drug Control Strategy: a national response to drug use. Washington, DC, US Government Printing Office, 1992a

Office of National Drug Control Policy: 1992 National Drug Control Strategy: a nation responds to drug use, budget summary. Washington, DC, US Government Printing Office, 1992b

Office of Technology Assessment: Smoking-Related Deaths and Financial Costs. US Congress, Staff Memorandum, September 1985

Parsons C, Kamenca A: Economic Impact of Drug Abuse in America. Bernard and Ellen Simonsen Fellowship Project. Los Angeles, University of Southern California, Graduate School of Business, 1992

Parsons C, Kamenca A: The Economic Cost of Alcohol Abuse in America: Bernard and Ellen Simonsen Fellowship Project. Los Angeles, University of Southern California, Graduate School of Business, 1993

Pickens RW, Leukefeld CG, Schuster CR: Improving Drug Abuse Treatment. National Institute on Drug Abuse Research Monograph No 106 (DHHS Publ No ADM-91-1754). Washington, DC, US Government Printing Office, 1991

Pincus HA, Fine T: The "anatomy" of research funding of mental illness and addictive disorders. Arch Gen Psychiatry 49:573–579, 1992

Plaut TFA (ed): Alcohol Problems: A Report to the Nation. New York, Oxford University Press, 1967

Reuter P: Hawks ascendant: the punitive trend of American drug policy. Daedalus 121:15–52, 1992

Rice DP, Kelman S, Miller LS, et al: The Economic Costs of Alcohol and Drug Abuse and Mental Illness: 1985. Report submitted to the Office of Financing and Coverage Policy of the Alcohol, Drug Abuse, and Mental Health Administration (DHHS Publ No ADM-90-1694). San Francisco, CA, University of California, Institute for Health and Aging, 1990

Saxe L, Dougherty D, Esty K, et al: The effectiveness and costs of alcoholism treatment. Washington, DC, Office of Technology Assessment, 1983

Sharfstein SS, Stoline AM, Goldman HH: Psychiatric care and health insurance reform. Am J Psychiatry 150:7–18, 1993

Smith E, Cloninger C, Bradford S: Predictors of mortality in alcoholic women: a prospective follow-up study. Alcohol Clin Exp Res 7:237–243, 1983

Smith DC, Mahoney JJ: McDonnell Douglas Corporation employee assistance program financial offset study, 1985–1988. Paper presented at annual conference of the Employee Assistance Professionals Association, Baltimore, MD, October 29–November 1, 1989

Substance Abuse and Mental Health Services Administration: Highlights from the 1991 National Drug and Alcoholism Treatment Unit Survey (NDATUS). Washington, DC, US Government Printing Office, 1992

Walsh DC, Hingson RW, Merrigan DM, et al: A randomized trial of treatment options for alcohol-abusing workers. N Engl J Med 325:775–782, 1991

Willenbring ML, Ridgley MS, Stinchfield R, et al: Application of case management in alcohol and drug dependence: matching techniques and populations (Contract No 89MF00933901D). Report to Homeless Demonstration and Evaluation Branch, National Institute of National Institute on Alcohol Abuse and Alcoholism. Rockville, MD, National Institute on Alcohol Abuse and Alcoholism, 1991

Zook CJ, Moore FD: High-cost users of medical care. N Engl J Med 302:996–1002, 1980

Chapter 4

Needs of the Addiction Treatment System

Having reviewed the extent and societal cost of addictive disorders and the present system of services available for treatment of addicted patients, we conclude this book with a discussion of the needs of this treatment system.

The current climate of consensus on the need for health system reform has brought with it a renewed interest in both primary care and prevention. This emphasis is particularly relevant to those health and social problems related to alcohol and drug use. Prevention through health education, brief interventions to promote the cessation of smoking and high-risk patterns of alcohol and other drug use, and screening followed by early intervention, are all appropriate and desirable activities in every primary care setting. However, few primary care practitioners or facilities are currently prepared to offer the full range of services needed to provide adequate treatment for the addictive disorders themselves, nor is it likely that primary caregivers will assume this function in the future. Specialty practitioners and facilities will remain essential to the care of this large and varied patient population, as will improved linkage with the primary care system.

Thus, the continued growth of the addiction treatment system into a universally accessible; gender-, age-, and culture-appropriate; and cost-effective service continuum must be part of the nation's overall health plan. To achieve this goal, several objectives will have to be met:

✦ *Improved screening and intervention*—Both primary care and specialty medical settings and other human service settings need improved systems for screening and intervention for persons with addictive disorders.

✦ *Improved linkage*—Linkage to primary care, specialty medical services, and other service systems must be strengthened.

✦ *Geographic uniformity*—The present system lacks geographic uniformity. Parts of the needed continuum of care are available in different areas, but specific service elements are simply unavailable in many communities.

✦ *Rational utilization*—Some existing facilities are underutilized for economic reasons, whereas others are disadvantaged by long waiting lists. A more equitable distribution of services is contingent on rational and stable financing mechanisms that would allow treatment in the most cost-effective setting in accordance with patient need.

✦ *Better fit between treatment modalities and patient needs*—There is a need to refine and develop the currently available treatment modalities and to match them more efficiently to patient need through research and the application of research findings to clinical practice.

✦ *Increased research into addictive diseases and their treatment*—There is a need for the development of new addiction treatments, both pharmacological and psychosocial, as well as better knowledge about the epidemiology, phenomenology, etiology, natural history, and treatment responsiveness of this group of disorders.

✦ *Clearer understanding of relationship between components of treatment system*—There is a need for better understanding of the service system, its components, their costs and benefits, the system's funding, and the effects of varying models of financing and cost control on the provision and effectiveness of addiction treatment.

✦ *Training*—Parallel to the above seven needs is the ongoing requirement for human resource development. There must be a national commitment to train both primary and specialty care health-human service professionals in prevention, identification, and early intervention.

Each of these needs is discussed below.

Identification, Screening, and Intervention

A number of screening methods are available to assist in the early recognition of addictive disorders. These range from sets of questions to include in a medical history, (e.g., the CAGE questions [Ewing 1984]) to structured questionnaires such as the Michigan Alcoholism Screening Test (Selzer 1971), the Drug Abuse Screening Test (Skinner 1982), the Alcohol Use Disorders Identification Test (AUDIT) (Saunders et al. 1993), and TWEAK (Russell et al. 1991), to chemical testing of breath, blood, and urine for substances of abuse. What is lacking in the present health care system is the provision of sufficient training, experience, incentives, and system requirements for the application of the available technology.

Practitioners in primary care settings, specialty practices (e.g., emergency medicine, obstetrics-gynecology, and orthopedic surgery), and general and psychiatric hospitals should all routinely screen for substance use disorders. As is discussed in Chapter 2, research studies have repeatedly demonstrated a high prevalence of addictive disorders in these settings. To promote such identification and early intervention, screening requirements should be widely included in practice guidelines and in systemwide review mechanisms. For example, screening and intervention could be included in accreditation criteria promulgated by the Joint Commission on Accreditation of Healthcare Organizations, state licensing agencies, Medicare peer review organizations, and other practice oversight bodies, as well as organizations that certify medical education programs. To satisfy these requirements, systems for routine screening, intervention, and referral would then be built into all relevant health systems. In 1991, the American Hospital Association recommended hospitalwide training and hospital policies that delineated systematic approaches to the identification of these disorders in all health care facilities. Model programs for use in general hospitals are also available (e.g., Lewis and Gordon 1983).

Similarly, both improved training and a systematic approach to screening and intervention are needed in other components of the human service system, including family and social welfare agencies, workplace-based employee benefit services, and the criminal justice system.

System Coordination and Linkage

To complement improvements in screening and intervention, improved linkage is required between primary care services, other components of the human service system, and the continuum of addiction treatment services in each community. Simplified referral systems should be developed, including coordination of services between specialty providers and increased involvement of the primary care provider in long-term follow-up.

Availability of Treatment

Although there has been much discussion of the concept of "treatment on demand," or, perhaps more accurately, "treatment as needed" (e.g., Legal Action Center 1991), the present system is far from achieving that ideal. As is discussed in Chapters 1 and 2, most individuals who currently receive help for addictive disorders do so outside of the specialty treatment system. The adequacy of this care is unknown. There is a need for better information about the nature and effectiveness of treatment of the substance use disorders outside of the addiction service system. However, there is also a clear need to continue to develop a network of services offering the full continuum of addiction treatment, as described in Chapter 2. The combination of an available continuum of care and the application of patient-treatment matching criteria will ensure a rational treatment system. Barriers that impede access to care (e.g., programs that are not culturally sensitive; programs that do not meet age-, gender-, or comorbidity-based patient needs; treatment that is inaccessible because of lack of insurance coverage or financial support) subvert such a system.

In addition, state alcohol and drug service oversight agencies, in collaboration with the Substance Abuse and Mental Health Services Administration, National Institute on Alcohol Abuse and Alcoholism (NIAAA), and National Institute on Drug Abuse (NIDA) should develop a common set of indicators for estimating the prevalence, service needs, and treatment costs of the substance use disorders, as recommended by the Institute of Medicine in its 1990 report. These needs-assessment methods are necessary to develop a uniform basis for service and fiscal planning. Planning should also be extended to 3- to 5-year cycles rather than on a year-by-year basis, as is now customary. Without a reasonable expectation of continuity of funding, publicly supported programs are seriously compromised in their staff recruitment and training as well as in their ability to perform adequate data collection and follow-up.

As the system continues to be developed, treatment facilities should be helped and encouraged to extend and adapt their programming to meet the needs of special populations, particularly homeless individuals, those from minority populations, women (including those who are pregnant or have small children), gay men and lesbians, adolescents, family members (including children of addicted parents), those with serious psychiatric co-morbidity, and those with serious physical problems (e.g., acquired immunodeficiency syndrome [AIDS]).

Treatment availability should be extended to fill the great unmet need in the criminal justice system (see Chapter 2). Improved access will continue to be needed in the military as well as health care systems provided for veterans (see Chapter 3). Particularly in facilities supported by the Department of Veterans Affairs, current statistics document large amounts of care provided for the complications of addictive disorders without equal attention to the underlying addiction. In addition, Indian Health Service programs could profit from a more complete continuum of care at the community level for individuals in need. Both alcohol dependence and fetal alcohol syndrome continue to present major problems for Native American and Alaskan Native communities, as do other drug-related problems.

Organization and Functioning of the Addiction Treatment System

Community Involvement

Involvement of community leaders and members is essential in the implementation of plans to improve and extend the continuum of addiction services. Community involvement not only will help prevent the "not in my backyard" attitude, but also will help recovering patients integrate into the community's workforce and civic activities. Existing programs should include community outreach activities (e.g., education programs, community services) wherever possible.

Coordination and Integration Into the Mainstream of Medical Care

The multiple service needs of the addicted population are discussed throughout this book. The addiction service system must strengthen its linkages to primary care and to the entire network of human services.

Although reaching the goal of integration into the mainstream of care will involve major economic changes (e.g., parity of insurance coverage with other medical care), other activities are also important. Collegial relationships, consultations, education, and training across the entire health care system will help promote integration. Psychiatrists specializing in addiction treatment can be particularly helpful in educating medical colleagues and dispelling negative attitudes toward addicted individuals and their families.

Improving Data Collection and Application

Improving the effectiveness of the current system will involve the more systematic application of current knowledge and the development of new knowledge, as discussed under the section "Improving Treatment System Components and Methods," below. Most addiction treatment programs currently lack the capacity to perform systematic data collection, including both initial information on patient status and follow-up data. Developing this capacity would require technical assistance in setting up sophisticated data systems and sufficient funding to support them. Systematic data collection is necessary to apply patient-treatment matching techniques as they continue to develop, to measure cost-effectiveness, and to improve overall knowledge of the system. An improved uniform data collection system would also allow more rational planning and resource allocation than is now possible.

Improving Utilization Review and Case Management Systems in Addiction Treatment

Problems encountered in the application of case management systems to addiction treatment are discussed in Chapter 3. To ensure that patient care is not compromised, regulation of utilization review organizations at the state or national level is needed (J. B. Cutler, American Psychiatric Association Division of Government Relations, unpublished letter to Mrs. Tipper Gore, May 1993), including the following requirements:

✦ Criteria for medical necessity and assignment to levels of care should be based on standards formulated by recognized medical organizations that are clinically and research based and then made available to providers and consumers.

✦ Decisions should be made by appropriately trained health care professionals. No denial of approval should be implemented without an evaluation of the case by a physician trained and qualified in addiction treatment.

✦ An appeals process should be included in any utilization review system.

✦ Confidentiality of patient information should be protected in conformity to federal and state regulations.

These minimum standards are needed to protect patients from inappropriate limitations on access to the addiction treatment that may mean the difference between life and death.

The President's Commission on Model State Drug Laws proposed a Model Managed Care Consumer Protection Act (1993) that embodied many of the provisions recommended by Cutler (J. B. Cutler, American Psychiatric Association Division of Government Relations, unpublished letter to Mrs. Tipper Gore, May 1993). The act also included a requirement for the use of established clinical assessment criteria and barred conflicts of interest by clinical decision makers.

Treatment System
Components and Methods

Application of Current Research

Much of the treatment-related research reported in scientific journals does not find its way into clinical practice in a timely way. An example is discussed under the section "Methadone and Other Opiate Maintenance Programs" (Chapter 2), in which inadequate dosages of methadone and inadequate lengths of maintenance treatment were found in surveys of program practices (D'Aunno and Vaughn 1991; Greenhouse 1991). The application of research findings to matching patient needs and treatment options and to other aspects of care will depend on adequate ongoing communication, training, and the incorporation of these research findings into the standards of licensing and other oversight bodies. The development of practice guidelines for addiction treatment by the American Psychiatric Association and others, incorporating research-generated knowledge, will facilitate this process (see also "Better Understanding of the Current Treatment System," below).

New Treatment Methods and Models

Improvements in the understanding of neurobiology, neuropharmacology, and the physiologic mechanisms of addiction bring with them opportunities to develop and study new pharmacological agents to assist in addiction treatment. Federal research support is appropriately directed toward this effort, and addiction psychiatrists can play an important role in the development and clinical testing of such treatments. However, research is needed in many other treatment areas as well. Improved treatment models and methods are needed for the special populations mentioned previously (i.e., homeless individuals, those from minority populations, women, gay men and lesbians, adolescents, elderly individuals, children of addicted parents, and patients with physical and psychiatric comorbidities). Research is needed to determine which of the multiple treatment methods offered by the program categories described in Chapter 2 work best with which populations. At present, program philosophy, staff availability and training, and clinical experience are often the major determinants of what treatments are offered. In many treatment programs patients are exposed to a wide variety of modalities in the expectation that they will derive some benefit from each or choose the one that is best for them.

Other research studies will also be critical to psychiatry's understanding of treatment. Results from the few studies reviewed in Chapter 3 have indicated that utilization management and cost-containment systems may have a significant effect on patient care. However, far more studies of the influences of delivery systems are necessary before these effects can be understood. Outcome data, in particular, should be correlated with delivery system and utilization data. Such studies can also provide useful feedback for program improvement.

Better Understanding of the Current Treatment System

Current nationwide surveys of the specialty addiction treatment system (e.g., the National Drug and Alcoholism Treatment Unit Survey) should be continued, improved, and extended to give a more complete and accurate picture of the size and characteristics of the current system. As changes in financing and the imposition of cost-control measures produce shifts in service utilization patterns, timely and accurate information will become even more critical to understanding the effects of such changes on patient care.

Support for the Addiction Treatment System

The two most important current policy issues affecting the future of support for addiction treatment are health system reform and strategy modifications in the national policy known as the "war on drugs." Related to these issues are the roles of current public and private insurance systems in supporting addiction treatment, and the sources, amounts, and roles of federal, state, and local direct funding of treatment programs.

Health System Reform

During the past few years, several proposals for reforming the health care system, either in whole or in part, have been introduced at both the state and federal levels. Health system reform presents an opportunity to integrate addiction treatment into the mainstream of medical care. The principles for reform proposed by the American Psychiatric Association (1993) would achieve this goal by including nondiscriminatory coverage for the prevention and treatment of addictive disorders on the same basis as all other medical care. These principles call for uniform benefits in all states and the extension of these benefits to all currently uninsured individuals without regard to previous illness. Any limitations on benefits, requirements for co-payments, or mandated deductibles for addiction services should be the same as are applied to any other illness. Catastrophic coverage should be provided for severely ill individuals, including those with severe addictions, with or without comorbid conditions. Utilization management systems should be applied in the same manner to all medical care and should support confidentiality and the quality of care.

The principles enunciated by the American Psychiatric Association (1993) are particularly important because they recognize that the addictive disorders are chronic in nature and cannot be successfully managed in an acute care model. Benefit limits such as one hospital admission per year, or one inpatient treatment allowed in a lifetime, ignore the fact that many addicted individuals undergo several treatment episodes, with intervening relapses, before long-term recovery is achieved. Furthermore, coverage for the entire continuum of care is essential. This will avoid the inappropriate utilization of more costly levels of care because of the unavailability of a more appropriate service of lower intensity.

Unfortunately, few of the reform proposals now under consideration meet these ideals of parity and the support of a complete continuum. Special limits continue to be proposed for psychiatric and addiction services, and some proposals fail to cover long-term care. Furthermore, Medicare, Medicaid, and other public and private insurance programs will remain separately funded and administered under many of the proposed models, perpetuating inequities in these systems. In addition, services to special populations, such as jail and prison inmates, are seldom included in reform systems. Some models also leave a significant proportion of the population uninsured.

Thus, whatever model of reform is ultimately adopted, the continued need for direct public funding of addiction services is almost certain. Proposals to redirect public funds currently appropriated to alcohol and drug abuse prevention and treatment to use in supporting general health system reform constitute a serious threat to the provision of adequate addiction treatment in the future. To the extent that the entire continuum of treatment services is not fully included within the basic benefit, measures must be taken to preserve the federal alcohol and drug block grant and state and local funding efforts.

In addition, many reform proposals contain financial incentives to limit benefits to the basic package. These include increased recipient contribution to the cost of insurance above the minimum benefit and taxing corporate funds used to purchase above-minimum policies for employees. These incentives make the inclusion of addiction treatment as a basic benefit even more critical, and highlight the need to preserve direct public funding of the safety net of services for patients who need more treatment than the benefit provides (Legal Action Center 1993).

While health care reform is being debated, efforts to improve benefits for the treatment of substance use disorders in current insurance plans should also continue. Collective bargaining and the enforcement of state mandates remain viable strategies to move the coverage for addiction closer to parity with other diseases. A 1993 report by the President's Commission on Model State Drug Laws, a bipartisan panel appointed in 1992, contained the recommendation that all states adopt legislation requiring that the full continuum of addiction treatment be provided by health insurance policies, health maintenance organizations, and state Medicaid programs. This statute should be adopted in all states.

The collection of accurate data about service utilization and costs under plans with different benefit structures is also an important priority. State and local decision makers need data to investigate the transfer of costs for the care of inadequately insured, addicted individuals to the public sector to make informed decisions about the need for insurance mandates and their costs. They also need data to understand the impact of utilization review–case management systems on access to care and on costs in the public sector.

Federal Spending in the "War on Drugs"

Much of the current federal spending on prevention and treatment of addictive disorders is subsumed under the rubric of *demand reduction* in the federal "war on drugs" (Office of National Drug Control Policy 1992; see also "Current System Financing," Chapter 3). In the past, the financing of this strategy has separated measures aimed against illicit drug use (hence, the so-called war on drugs) from measures aimed at preventing and treating other addiction-related problems, such as smoking-related diseases, alcohol dependence, alcohol-related highway and other accidents, fetal alcohol syndrome, and alcohol-related violence. Funds for research by NIDA are included in the national drug strategy, whereas research funds appropriated to NIAAA for alcohol-related research are not. Although the history of the national drug strategy makes the separation of illegal drug problems from other addiction problems understandable, many field representatives argue that this strategy ignores the fact that often problems related to tobacco and alcohol are intertwined with problems involving illegal drugs. In terms of social costs, separation of prevention and treatment for these two categories of drugs (i.e., alcohol as a legal drug versus other psychoactive substances as illegal drugs) makes little sense. Extending federal level planning and coordination activities to the consideration of problems related to all drugs of abuse would improve the effectiveness and efficiency of the federal effort.

A second proposal to alter the current federal strategy would be to reapportion federal funds between supply reduction and demand reduction efforts. Over the past 12 years, prevention, treatment, and research (i.e., demand reduction) have accounted for only 20%–30% of total federal funds expended on drug-related problems. A shift to a 50%-50% allocation of funds would make sufficient funds available to expand treatment availability, improve existing treatment (including improvements in staffing, training, and data collection), provide services in the criminal justice system, expand research into treatment effectiveness and matching between patient needs and treatment options, and improve prevention (Legal Action Center 1991).

In a study done by the Drug Policy Research Center of the Rand Corporation, Rydell and Everingham (1994) supported the recommendation that increased resources be spent on treatment. Confining themselves to cocaine, the authors analyzed the relative cost-effectiveness of investing federal dollars in control of cocaine supply within the source country, interdiction, domestic enforcement, and treatment. They estimated that, to decrease the total cocaine consumption in the United States by 1%, an additional $34 million would have to be invested in addiction treatment. Achieving that same 1% reduction through supply reduction efforts would require that $783 million be spent for additional source-country control, $366 million for interdiction, or $246 million for domestic enforcement. Thus, the least costly supply reduction strategy would cost 7.3 times as much as an investment in treatment for an equivalent effect. Although similar estimates have not been made for other drugs such as heroin or marijuana, the Rand study provides forceful support for a reallocation of federal antidrug funding.

A 1993 report from the General Accounting Office reviewed a wide range of alternative approaches to the present federal drug control strategy. The resulting suggested alternatives to the current funding formula would rely less heavily on enforcement but would still preserve the strategic focus on illegal drugs.

Additional recommendations have been made by the National Association of State Alcohol and Drug Abuse Directors (NASADAD) in its 1992 National Drug Control Policy White Paper. In the paper, it was suggested that the war metaphor, as reflected in the framing of the national strategy as a "war on drugs," was not the most appropriate mind-set for the social policy needed to deal with the country's addiction problems. Rather than preserving the division between strategies to control alcohol and tobacco problems and those aimed at illegal drugs, NASADAD recommended a wider and more health-focused approach, including a suggestion that the term war on drugs be discarded in favor of a more positive approach framed in positive language. It is noteworthy that the 1993 Interim National Drug Control Strategy, unlike previous strategy documents, did not stress the analogy of a war. Instead the language used discusses "acknowledging drug abuse as a public health problem" (Office of National Drug Control Policy 1993, p. 2). However, even in that report, an alcohol and tobacco control strategy is still not integrated with that related to illegal drugs.

State and Local Funding

As discussed in Chapter 3, state and local funding has replaced federal funding as the predominant source of public support for the community-based network of addiction treatment programs. This funding source will continue to play a vital role in the support of addiction programs after the implementation of health system reform. At the very least, state and local funds will be called on to support the vocational, educational, and other rehabilitative services needed by individuals recovering from an addiction and the housing, transportation, and child care services needed to make treatment accessible to disadvantaged populations. These funds will also be called on to provide services in jails and prisons.

More likely, as discussed above, the benefits provided by health system reform will not include nondiscriminatory coverage of the entire continuum of addiction treatment. Long-term care, such as that provided by methadone maintenance programs, therapeutic communities, and community residences may not be included. Individuals who have severe and persistent disease, particularly those with significant comorbid disorders, may require intensive long-term services not provided by the standard benefit. It is critical to the care of addicted individuals and their families that public funds continue to be allocated to provide for their treatment. Significant increases in federal, state, and local direct funding are needed immediately, even before health system reform plans are legislated, as any health reform plan adopted will be phased in over several years. The present financial status of the publicly funded system of community-based addiction treatment programs has been challenged by the failure of federal, state, and local appropriations to keep up with inflation (Leukefeld et al. 1991). These programs, in many localities, need an infusion of funds just to meet the present demand.

Medicare and Medicaid

Because Medicare is currently and will remain an important source of support for addiction treatment for its beneficiaries, the Medicare program should continue to be altered to meet the needs of those with substance use disorders. The lifetime limit of 190 days of hospital care should be dropped because it is not also applied to general medical care. In addition, refinement of the diagnosis-related group system to account for different types of substance use disorders and different levels of severity would be helpful.

Medicare Part B should be revised to remove the inequities in reimbursement based on the resource-based relative value scale. In addition, parity of benefits for the treatment of psychiatric and substance use disorders with payment for all other illnesses should be a guiding principle.

The Medicaid system, with its shared federal and state funding, is a support mechanism that has been underutilized for the treatment of addictive disorders (Gerstein and Harwood 1990). As discussed in Chapter 3, although Medicaid recipients with substance use disorders consume a disproportionate share of resources, little is spent on direct treatment of the addiction itself (Center on Addiction and Substance Abuse 1993). To remedy this situation, the Institute of Medicine made several recommendations (Gerstein and Harwood 1990). The most important among these was that addiction treatment be included within the federally mandated benefits provided for all recipients. The institute also recommended a system of public utilization management to ensure access to appropriate treatment. An additional sorely needed change is lifting the current institution for mental disorder restriction for Medicaid recipients between ages 22 and 65 years (see discussion of Medicaid in Chapter 3). This exclusion was originally instituted to preclude Medicaid support for custodial care. This consideration is totally inappropriate to inpatient treatment for substance use disorders. Appropriate treatment of addictive disorders among Medicaid recipients would produce cost savings within the general health Medic-aid budget to offset, in whole or in part, the additional expenditure once this exclusion was removed.

A measure placed before Congress in 1991 (the Medicaid Substance Abuse Treatment Act) proposed to remove part of the present Medicaid restriction by allowing the use of federal Medicaid funds to reimburse specialized residential care for pregnant and postpartum women and their children for up to 1 year (National Council on Alcoholism and Drug Dependence 1992). This bill is an important step toward making Medicaid the viable source of addiction treatment support it could become. The President's Commission on Model State Drug Laws (1993) recommended that the full continuum of addiction treatment be covered in each state's Medicaid plan. The commission also proposed the Model Early and Peri-odic Screening, Diagnosis and Treatment (EPSDT) Services Act. In this proposal, each state is encouraged to take advantage of the 1989 federal legislation that allowed the inclusion of alcohol and other drug screening, counseling, and treatment among the federally participating EPSDT ser-vices available to children and adolescents in the Medicaid program. Both of these proposed laws should be adopted by the states.

Potential Sources of Public Funding

Additional public funds to support the treatment of substance use disorders could be derived from increases in the taxes levied on tobacco products and alcoholic beverages. These taxes are paid predominantly by the heaviest users, who also contribute most to societal cost.

Additional funds could also be derived by redirecting resources cur-rently used for supply reduction in the war on drugs (General Accounting Office 1993; National Association of State Alcohol and Drug Abuse Direc-tors 1992; Legal Action Center 1991; Office of National Drug Control Policy 1992) and from asset forfeiture funds, most of which are currently devoted to law enforcement (Legal Action Center 1991).

Research Needs

Throughout the discussion of the addiction treatment system in this book, the need for a better understanding of substance use disorders, including their causes, epidemiology, cost to society, natural history (particularly in special populations), and their treatment, has been stressed. The need for better understanding of treatment processes, effectiveness, costs versus benefits, and patient-treatment matching has also been discussed. Equally needed to enable rational development of the treatment system are better data on the economics of delivery systems and cost control factors as they relate to patient care and outcome.

As discussed in Chapter 3, the federal research institutes—NIDA and NIAAA—support a larger proportion of the total national research effort in substance use disorders than do other bodies of the National Institutes of Health for their special branches of medicine. NIDA and NIAAA are already unable to fund many important studies. They need both an increase in total funding and a stability of year-to-year funding so that their research program planning can be more rational.

In addition, other sources for research funds, including private industry and charitable foundations, should be educated about the social costs of the substance use disorders and be encouraged to increase their interest in the area.

At the same time, there is a need for better dissemination of current research, both to clinicians and program administrators on one hand and to public policy makers on the other. Barriers to dissemination include a lack of sufficient forums for discussion between researchers, clinicians, and policy makers; inadequate resources for continuing education and training at the program level; relative inaccessibility of professional journals to front-line staff; and a lack of interest in and commitment to research by some providers (New York State Office of Alcoholism and Substance Abuse Services 1993). All of these factors can be improved by better communication and increased training resources.

Training Needs

The need for improved training in the prevention and treatment of substance use disorders has already been mentioned. Health and human service practitioners at all levels require better preparation to screen, intervene with, and refer those in need of treatment. Treatment providers and administrators need better mastery of current research findings. Policy makers need a better grasp of the nature and extent of the substance use disorders and the value and cost of treatment.

To fulfill these training needs, especially within the medical education system, support for fellowships in addiction psychiatry and other areas of addiction medicine are required. A stable funding base for addiction psychiatry fellowships will be needed to support psychiatrists wishing to take the examination for added qualifications in addiction psychiatry, offered by the American Board of Psychiatry and Neurology since 1993. These psychiatrists will in turn play an increasing role as teachers, consultants, and leaders in the field.

Faculty development support will also be necessary to prepare an adequate supply of younger faculty so that education about addictive disorders may be taught within mainstream medical education. Without strong leadership, teaching about these disorders is likely to lose out in the competition for teaching time within the curriculum. Federal programs like the Career Teachers Program sponsored by NIDA and NIAAA in the 1970s and early 1980s should be reestablished to help develop the academic leadership needed within medical education. An expansion of the recently funded addiction training centers sponsored by the Center for Substance Abuse Treatment will help to address the need for trained professionals.

Other professional training institutions have similar needs for faculty development support. Adequate training of all health professionals in addiction will be necessary for the establishment of the full range of addiction services.

References

American Hospital Association: Caring for Patients With Alcohol and Other Drug Problems. Chicago, IL, American Hospital Association, 1991

American Psychiatric Association: Policy statement on national health care reform. Psychiatric News 28(19):7, 1993

Center on Addiction and Substance Abuse: The Cost of Substance Abuse to America's Health Care System, Report 1: Medicaid Hospital Costs, A CASA Report. New York, Center on Addiction and Substance Abuse at Columbia University, 1993

D'Aunno T, Vaughn TE: Variations in methadone treatment practices. JAMA 267:253–258, 1991

Ewing JA: Detecting alcoholism: the CAGE questionnaire. JAMA 252:1905–1907, 1984

General Accounting Office: Confronting the Drug Problem: Debate Persists on Enforcement and Alternative Approaches (Publ GAO/GGD-93-82). Washington, DC, General Accounting Office, 1993

Gerstein DR, Harwood HJ (eds): Treating Drug Problems, Vol 1. Washington, DC, National Academy Press, 1990

Greenhouse CM: Study finds methadone treatment practices vary widely in effectiveness. NIDA Notes 7:1–5, 1991

Institute of Medicine: Broadening the Base of Treatment for Alcohol Problems. Washington, DC, American Psychiatric Press, 1990

Legal Action Center: Blueprint for a New and Effective National Drug and Alcohol Strategy. New York, Legal Action Center, 1991

Legal Action Center: Position Paper on the Coverage of Substance Abuse Treatment in the American Health Security Act. New York, Legal Action Center, 1993

Leukefeld CG, Pickens RW, Schuster CR: Improving drug abuse treatment: recommendations for research and practice. NIDA Research Monograph Series 106 (DHHS Publ No ADM-91-1754). Washington, DC, US Government Printing Office, 1991

Lewis D, Gordon AJ: Alcoholism in the general hospital: the Roger Williams intervention program. Bull N Y Acad Med 59:181–197, 1983

National Association of State Alcohol and Drug Abuse Directors: National Drug Control White Paper—Alcohol and Other Drug Problems: Coordination and Cross-Cutting Solutions. Washington, DC, National Association of State Alcohol and Drug Abuse Directors, 1992

National Council on Alcoholism and Drug Dependence: Insurance Coverage for Alcoholism and Drug Treatment: An Activist's Guide for Making Your Voice Heard in the Federal Health Care Reform Debate. Washington, DC, National Council on Alcoholism and Drug Dependence, 1992

New York State Office of Alcoholism and Substance Abuse Services: Anti-Drug Abuse Council Research Forum: Summary Report. Albany, NY, New York State Office of Alcoholism and Substance Abuse Services, 1993

Office of National Drug Control Strategy: National Drug Control Policy: A National Response to Drug Use. Washington, DC, US Government Printing Office, 1992

Office of National Drug Control Policy: Breaking the Cycle of Drug Abuse: 1993 Interim National Drug Control Strategy. Washington, DC, US Government Printing Office, 1993

President's Commission on Model State Drug Laws: Executive Summary. Washington, DC, US Government Printing Office, 1993

Russell M, Martier SS, Sokol RJ: Screening for pregnancy risk-drinking: tweaking the tests. Alcohol Clin Exp Res 15:268, 1991

Rydell PC, Everingham SS: Controlling Cocaine: Supply Versus Demand Programs. Santa Monica, CA, RAND Corporation, 1994

Saunders JB, Aasland OG, Amundsen A, et al: Alcohol consumption and related problems among primary health care patients: WHO Collaborative Project on Early Detection of Persons With Harmful Alcohol Consumption—I. Addiction 88:349–362, 1993

Selzer ML: The Michigan Alcoholism Screening Test: the quest for a new diagnostic instrument. Am J Psychiatry 127:89–94, 1971

Skinner HA: The Drug Abuse Screening Test (DAST). Addictive Behaviors 7:363–371, 1982

Chapter 5

Conclusion

In this report, we have tried to provide a picture of the development and current status of services for addicted patients. A review of the history of the addiction treatment system reveals that this service system was developed relatively recently compared with other health care systems. In addition, because of the peculiarities of its financing, the system has not yet developed a full continuum of treatment services for the majority of persons in need. The growth of the system has led to a two-tier, public-private dichotomy, along with uneven utilization of resources and a skewed geographical distribution. Remedies are available within the present system if society has the will and ability to establish and manage adequate treatment for these disorders. In addition, reform of the health care system at the state and national levels present opportunities to bring these services into the mainstream of medical care with a stable funding base.

We have suggested some steps that can be taken to improve the nation's response to its widespread and devastating addiction problems. Psychiatrists, as ideally suited providers and advocates, should increase their efforts and knowledge, both as individuals and jointly with others interested in health and welfare, to influence state and national policy to reach these goals.

Index